Praise for

Empower Yourself Against Racial and Cultural Stress

"This book made me aware of stress and anxiety that I didn't realize I had, but also gave me ways to release it. I absolutely loved the Relationship and Community Map."

—Daysia B., Detroit, Michigan

"This book opened my eyes to the ways cultural stressors have shaped not only how I see the world but also how I see myself. For example, the BEAT diagram taught me how to check in with myself not just emotionally, but physically and mentally too, and to approach those feelings with curiosity instead of judgment. The combination of reflection and action is what makes this book stand out."

—Mariah P., Louisville, Kentucky

"As an African American college student on the verge of entering the corporate world, I know I'll be surrounded by people who don't look like me, and I will be forced to prove myself time and time again. The coping practices in this book really resonate with me."

—Kaliyah J., Indianapolis, Indiana

"It was eye-opening for me to share this book with my son and hear his perspectives on the challenges he knows he will face as a young adult Black male. We've talked about these issues many times, but the book was very helpful in organizing and directing the conversation."

—Darlene D., Dayton, Ohio

"This book helped me confront some feelings and identity issues I've been dealing with for a while. I like that Dr. DeLapp offers an abundance of solutions, versus just explaining the causes of stress."

—Shelby J., Lexington, Kentucky

"This workbook gives you concrete strategies for both tackling stress and understanding yourself better amid society's varied racial challenges. Most exciting is the choose-your-own-path format, giving you extensive examples and options to help customize your journey through the book."

—Riana Elyse Anderson, PhD, School of Social Work, Columbia University

"Dr. DeLapp addresses the unique stresses you face as a young person of color and provides evidence-based tools to help navigate them. I appreciate the interactive components, empowering stories, and practical guidance for dealing with difficult situations. An invaluable resource."

—Erlanger A. Turner, PhD, author of *Raising Resilient Black Kids*

"This 'must-have' book is jam-packed with evidence-based, practical strategies. Through relatable stories and engaging worksheets and activities, Dr. DeLapp draws on extensive personal and professional experience to help you build your own 'coping toolkit.'"

—Phyllis L. Fagell, LCPC, author of *Middle School Matters* and *Middle School Superpowers*

"This insightful, affirming book is much needed and long overdue. Dr. DeLapp empowers you not only to build coping skills, but also to grow, heal, and overcome racial challenges."

—Monnica T. Williams, PhD, ABPP, School of Psychology, University of Ottawa, Canada

"Dr. DeLapp is an expert on treatment considerations for racism-related stress. He has created a highly interactive, engaging book with a treasure trove of practical tools derived from CBT, DBT, ACT, CFT, and other evidence-based approaches."

—Simon A. Rego, PsyD, ABPP, coauthor of *The CBT Workbook for Mental Health*

Empower Yourself Against Racial and Cultural Stress

EMPOWER YOURSELF AGAINST RACIAL AND CULTURAL STRESS

Using Skills from the REACH Program to Cope, Heal, and Thrive

Ryan C. T. DeLapp, PhD

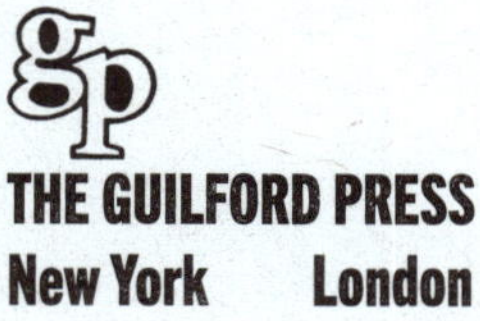

THE GUILFORD PRESS
New York London

A Division of Guilford Publications, Inc.
www.guilford.com

The information in this volume is not intended as a substitute for consultation with healthcare professionals. Each individual's health concerns should be evaluated by a qualified professional.

Printed in the United States of America

Last digit is print number: 9 8 7 6 5 4 3 2 1

Library of Congress Cataloging-in-Publication Data is available from the publisher.

ISBN 978-1-4625-5308-2

Contents

Purchasers of this book can download and print worksheets at *www.guilford.com/delapp-forms* for personal use or use with clients (see copyright page for details).

Acknowledgments

So many people have contributed to the inception, execution, and completion of this labor of love. I want to first thank my amazing wife for her love and support during the writing of this book. Thanks for being my expert sounding board and for helping me remain grounded. To my parents, thank you for being the world's greatest cheerleaders. Your unrelenting encouragement to stay the course and trust God's plan for this project were invaluable. To my sister, thank you for contributing your honest teenage perspectives on the book's material. It feels good to know this book is "sister approved"! To my extended family (both living and deceased), thank you for helping me grow a deep love and appreciation for my racial and cultural background. To my many mentors, thank you for helping me see and trust my potential as an innovator within the mental health field. To my Guilford Press publishing team, I am grateful for the opportunity and platform to share my work via this book. And special shout-out to my wonderfully gifted editor, Christine Benton—thank you for helping me refine the message of this book. To the Ross Center, thank you for acknowledging the importance of the Racial, Ethnic, and Cultural Healing (REACH) program and its workbook and helping me expand the "reach" of my clinical practice. To my community partners, thank you for inviting me into your community spaces and allowing me to serve your young people. And, most importantly, to the many participants in the REACH program over the years, I am indebted to you all. Thank you for trusting me and my work as an added resource in your life's journey.

Introduction

Welcome to This Workbook

Welcome! If you identify as a person of color, this book can help you learn to cope with moments of feeling judged unfairly, mistreated, or denied opportunities based on your racial and cultural background. In this book, such moments are called **culturally stressful events.** Culturally stressful moments can cause pain and rob you of a sense of empowerment when they occur. And, if left unaddressed, their impact can also build over time. Maybe you've been unsure about how to respond to an insensitive comment. Or you haven't known how to address being denied an opportunity because of who you are. Or possibly you have been confused about exactly what you were feeling but can tell something feels emotionally off. This book is designed to help you build awareness of how such incidents are affecting you and then identify a course of action for navigating those impacts. It is based on the skills offered in the Racial, Ethnic, and Cultural Healing (REACH) program and uses a workbook format to help you learn and use those skills to feel more empowered in your daily life. With this book you will learn to practice **empowered coping** through three steps:

1. **Clarify the impacts of cultural stress:** The first step is to notice that there are three impacts of culturally stressful events—uncomfortable emotions that are hard to manage (*emotional stress*), feeling as if you do not have control over the situation (*agency stress*), and negative, critical thoughts about your racial and cultural background (*identity stress*). This book will help you build skills to stay aware of each impact—the foundation for choosing an empowering response to the culturally stressful events that occur in your relationships or community.

2. **Think of what you *can* do:** Once you are able to notice and acknowledge culturally stressful events, you can identify what remains within your power and

control to address them. We all are tasked with developing a coping toolkit for life's stresses. By completing this book, you will be introduced to (or possibly reminded of) what you *can* do when faced with cultural stress.

3. **Make empowered coping decisions:** Culturally stressful situations can throw us off balance even when we've prepared by building and practicing skills. One day it may seem that the best coping strategy is to confront the person causing you cultural stress. The next day you may feel it's better to save your energy and resist urges to be confrontational. Empowered coping comes from discovering your own answers to questions like "What coping decisions are best for me in this moment?" and "What's going to serve me best in the future?" These are tough decisions for all, and there is rarely one perfect choice. But this workbook will help you navigate difficult situations in the best possible way for you.

MEETING YOUR EMPOWERED NAVIGATORS

We all gain ideas for empowered coping from the people around us. Swapping stories, sharing lessons learned, and observing others' actions can give us new and creative ways to navigate the obstacles created by cultural stress. In fact, leading therapy groups with teens and young adults revealed to me how powerful it can be to have a trusted community of people there to help you. In an effort to simulate this community, I've included the stories of Greg, Amia, and Jamal, who I refer to as navigators, to accompany you on your journey toward empowered coping. Hopefully at least one of these three fictional characters will resonate with your own experiences and help you envision how you might use the skills you learn in this workbook on your own journey.

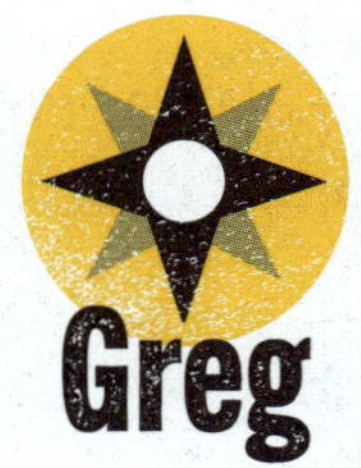

Greg is an 18-year-old Latino who lives with his parents and two younger sisters in a small city. He has grown up in a culturally diverse neighborhood, and is often surrounded by peers who look and sound just like him. Though once a thriving and exciting place to live, Greg's community is now riddled with violence and beaten down by poverty—often causing Greg and his family to avoid leaving or even hanging out in front of their home. From an early age, Greg has wanted to find some way to leave his community. Viewing college as his ticket out has motivated him to try his best in school and sports. But now, as he watches local kids dropping out or just hanging around the neighborhood, he finds himself wondering, "Is college even for someone like me?" or "Will I ever be able to leave?" And, during his time in high school, Greg has dreamed of attending a different school. He hoped this would have allowed him to be with people who share his love for learning and don't make him feel less-than for wanting to better himself.

He's tired of being called hurtful names for doing his best to listen to his teachers and for answering questions correctly in class. We are meeting Greg in his senior year as he begins to figure out what he wants to do after high school. Greg is looking to make a plan for next year that offers him a new, safer normal and allows him to honor his parents, who sacrificed their own dreams to create new opportunities for him and his sisters.

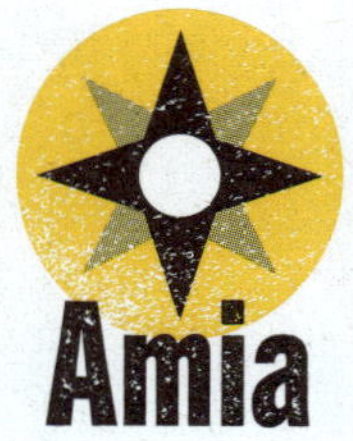

Amia, age 16, immigrated to the United States with her family two years ago. Her parents chose to leave the Middle East to escape political unrest and find better education opportunities for Amia and her siblings. When they moved to the United States, Amia and her family had yet to learn English and relied on extended family members who had been in the United States for several years to find their way. Amia struggled to understand her teachers and classmates in her new school until her fluency in English improved. It was at this time that she learned how much her peers were teasing her about her accent, skin color, and Islamic faith. These comments hurt Amia deeply, but she felt powerless to do anything about them. She was still struggling to make close friendships, her teachers did not seem able to stop the teasing she reported, and her parents were unsure how to advocate for her. Amia's anxiety has led her to skip school to avoid the relentless teasing. We are meeting Amia at a time when she feels very overwhelmed by the cultural stress within her school and she is unsure what to do.

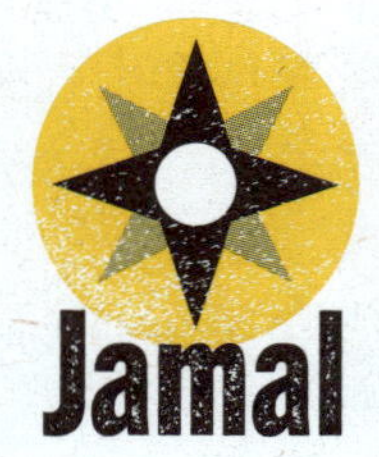

Jamal, 23 and Black, was raised in the American South in a very religious family and strongly identifies with his Christian faith. Jamal excelled academically during grade school and in college, as he was taught that the path to excellence for a Black man is a good education. Jamal had to leave friends and family behind in his predominantly Black community to attend prestigious schools elsewhere. College didn't change the fact that he was often the only Black student in his classes. A full scholarship enabled him to access a good higher education, but he found himself surrounded by people who did not look like him or share many of his interests. Jamal appreciates his Black identity but finds himself feeling as if he does not belong in most social spaces. He feels that he was never truly accepted within his mostly non-Black academic spaces and has felt a disconnect from his peers when attending predominantly Black community events. We are meeting Jamal in the year right after he has finished college. He is a young, well-educated professional who is learning to navigate corporate America as a Black man while also seeking to find peer relationships where he feels more accepted.

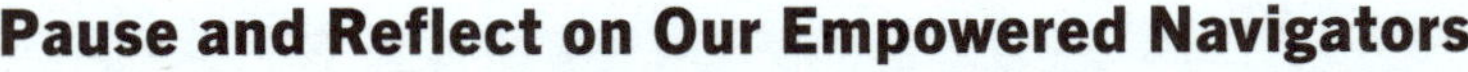

Pause and Reflect on Our Empowered Navigators

In this workbook you will have the opportunity to reflect on your experience and choose your own path to coping. By tapping into your own experiences of cultural stress, you'll be able to learn and grow—recapturing your power to determine your own life course. Please take the time to pause and carefully think through the reflection questions throughout the book so you can deepen your ability to understand and use the information in each chapter. Here's a chance to try it right now. (You can record your answers in a journal if you find there isn't enough space provided in this workbook to fit your responses, or, if you're using this book in a group setting, the leader might want to use the questions to start a discussion.)

Did you feel a connection with some aspects of the navigators' stories you just read? Take a few moments to consider which parts of their experiences were most relatable to yours and record your answers below.

Have you ever had a thought like Jamal's that he isn't accepted by people around him? If so, who were you around when you had such thoughts?

Have you ever experienced intense emotions, such as when Amia described feeling overwhelmed by cultural stress in her school? If so, what kinds of emotions have you felt?

Have you lived in a community like Greg's and felt your dreams weren't supported or you didn't have the resources needed to get where you wanted to go in life? If so, which of your dreams or goals have you felt that your surroundings do not support?

Was there anything else that stood out to you about any of the navigators' stories?

USING THIS WORKBOOK

Building empowered coping involves building both understanding and skills, using the worksheets and other activities provided in the rest of this book. Each exercise or activity begins with an overview of the steps involved. Then you'll read an example from one of our navigators. Finally, you'll be given instructions and worksheets to use toward building that skill. All of the worksheets in this book are available at *www.guilford.com/delapp-forms*. If you don't want to fill them out directly in the book, or you need more space, you can download and print the forms and fill them in separately.

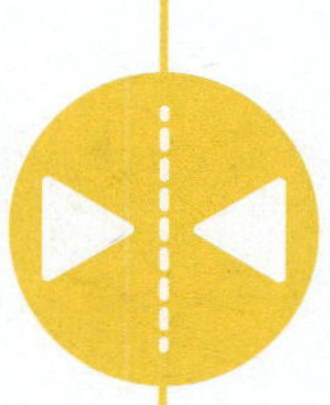

Introduction: Recap and Reflect

You have just completed the introduction to the this workbook. Congrats! The topic of cultural stress can be difficult, sensitive, and challenging, but I feel so much gratitude for being able to join you on this journey through the workbook. At the conclusion of each chapter moving forward, you'll find a "Recap and Reflect" section that summarizes the main takeaways and offers you a final reflection opportunity to help you prepare to move ahead.

RECAP

- **Culturally stressful events** describe the moments when we question whether we have been or might be unfairly judged, mistreated, or denied an opportunity due to our racial and cultural background.
- In this workbook, we will discuss three ways cultural stress can impact our lives—**emotional stress, agency stress,** and **identity stress.**
- This workbook is designed to help you strengthen your ability to engage in **empowered coping,** which includes (1) clarifying how cultural stress is impacting you, (2) identifying what you can do to cope with its impacts, and (3) making the most empowered coping decision for you in a given moment.

REFLECT

Can you find your own workbook navigators? (Use the worksheet on page 6 to list them.) Having supportive people (or even just one) to consult along your journey can help you learn more about your own experiences, better understand the impacts of cultural stress, and find ways to make empowered coping decisions when faced with culturally stressful experiences. These individuals could be family, friends, teachers, coaches, mentors, or health professionals—anyone who:

- Has a racial or cultural background similar to yours
- Might complete this workbook with you
- Will feel comfortable talking to about your reactions to the workbook materials

My Workbook Navigators

Name	Relationship to you	Why you chose them as navigators

PART ONE

Getting Started

1 What Does Being a Person of Color Mean to Me?

This workbook is intended for teens and young adults who identify themselves as *persons of color* (POCs), defined in this workbook as those who have certain lived experiences due to their shared *racial and cultural backgrounds.* In this chapter, you'll have the opportunity to explore what being a POC means to you.

WHAT DO WE MEAN BY RACIAL AND CULTURAL BACKGROUND?

Your **racial background** is the racial category that you or others place you in based on your physical characteristics—skin color, hair type, facial features, body type, and so forth. For some people, their racial category has little meaning in their daily life. For many, however, their racial category carries great significance, often due to the meaning society has attributed to certain physical characteristics. For example, people with lighter skin colors, like White-presenting individuals, have historically been seen as more beautiful, more intelligent, and less dangerous than those with darker skin. Such biases can be very hurtful and can impact the daily lives of people from certain racial backgrounds. So, the term *POC* can be used to capture the shared experience of people who face judgment, mistreatment, and denied opportunities because of their physical characteristics.

Interestingly, physical characteristics alone don't fully capture what it can mean to identify as a POC. Worldwide, groups of people with a variety of skin colors identify as POCs. This is where the term *culture* comes into the picture. Your **cultural background** refers to the customs, traditions, interests, languages, and general daily experiences unique to POCs. These cultural experiences can include musical, dance, food, and religious traditions shared and celebrated by POCs. And just as racial background can lead to culturally stressful events, cultural experiences viewed as "not normal" or "inferior" can also result in unfair judgment, mistreatment, and denied opportunity.

Pause and Reflect on the Term *Person of Color*

Teens and young adults I've spoken with have mixed feelings about the use of this term. Some find POC to be a helpful way to acknowledge how their experiences in certain settings are different from those of their White peers and colleagues. Others find this term too broad and an inappropriate label for their experience. Please take a few moments to think about your reactions to this term and its use in the community spaces you are in and record your thoughts below.

Where have you heard the terms *person of color* or *POC* used?

What are your thoughts and feelings about the term *person of color?*

Would you add to or change the definition of this term provided above? If yes, what would you add or change? If no, what about the definition provided above connects with your experience?

HOW TO COMPLETE THE "WHO AM I?" DIAGRAM

How do you see yourself as a POC? Your work toward using empowered coping starts with gaining an understanding of how your racial and cultural background fits into your overall sense of who you are. You will be asked to think about how your identities ("I am"), strengths ("I can do"), interests ("I like to do"), and values ("I care about") in the Who Am I? diagram are connected with your racial and cultural background.

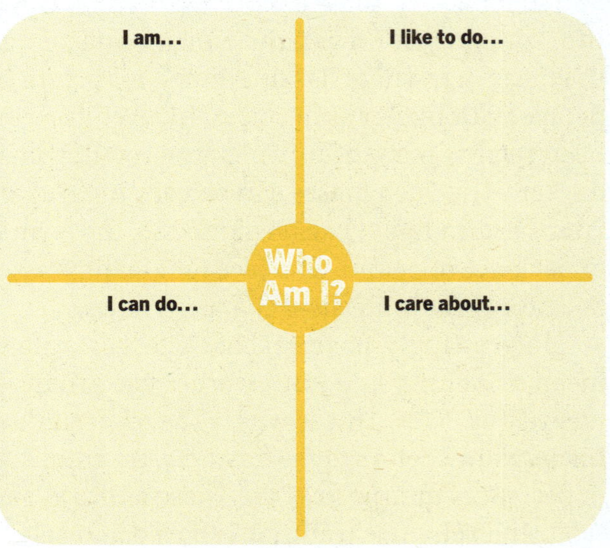

"I AM": WHAT ARE YOUR IDENTITIES?

Identity describes the personal traits and characteristics that we consider to be the most defining parts of who we are. These parts of ourselves are often captured by "I am" statements, like I am Black, I am Asian American, or I am Latina. Use the prompts below to help you complete this part of the Who Am I? diagram on page 14. And, if you have any difficulty knowing how to best represent your identities, consider completing this portion of the chapter with one of your workbook navigators (the people you listed on page 6).

1. **What is your racial/ethnic identity?** Your racial/ethnic identity is rooted in your family's lineage and story. You may enjoy the privilege of being able to trace your family's story for generations and highlight countries of origin and immigration histories. Or it may be very difficult for you to trace your roots. Use the lists on the next page to check off the categories with which you identify. There is space to add any that are not yet listed.

2. **What are your intersecting identities?** In addition to your racial/ethnic identity, you may feel that other parts of your identity are important to you. Check off any of the other categories on page 13 that feel like important parts of your identity to acknowledge.

3. **Fill in your Who Am I? diagram.** Now, list the identities that you feel are most important to you—including the labels you used to describe your racial and cultural background—in your **Who Am I? diagram** on page 14.

Pause and Reflect on Your Identities

Our identities have a greater meaning than simply checking a box on a form. Take a moment to think about the significance of the boxes you checked—specifically reflecting on how they define what being a POC means to you. Record your thoughts below.

When did you first begin identifying yourself using the labels you selected in the **racial and ethnic identities** part of this exercise?

Who has supported your discovery of these racial and ethnic identities? A family member, friend, teacher, or someone from another part of your community?

Are your racial and ethnic identities *visible* and *noticeable* to others? If yes, how does it feel when others acknowledge this part of your Who Am I? diagram? If no, how does it feel when others ignore, confuse, or do not acknowledge these identities?

(continue reflecting on your identities on page 15)

My Racial/Ethnic Identity

☐ **American Indian, Native American, or Alaska Native**

If selected, specify tribe:

☐ Navajo Nation
☐ Blackfeet Tribe
☐ Mayan
☐ Aztec
☐ Native Village of Barrow Inupiat Traditional Government
☐ Tlingit
☐ Unsure
☐ Other:

☐ **Asian**

If selected, are you:

☐ Cambodian
☐ Chinese
☐ Filipino
☐ Indian
☐ Japanese
☐ Korean
☐ Pakistani
☐ Thai
☐ Vietnamese
☐ Unsure
☐ Other Asian not listed (please describe):

☐ **Black or African American**

If selected, are you:

☐ African American
☐ Ethiopian
☐ Ghanaian
☐ Haitian
☐ Jamaican
☐ Nigerian
☐ Somali
☐ South African
☐ Kenyan
☐ Ugandan
☐ Unsure
☐ Other Black not listed (please describe):

☐ **Hispanic, Latino/a/x, or Spanish origin**

If selected, are you:

☐ Colombian
☐ Cuban
☐ Dominican
☐ Ecuadorian
☐ Guatemalan
☐ Mexican, Mexican American, or Chicano
☐ Salvadoran
☐ Puerto Rican
☐ Honduran
☐ Venezuelan
☐ Unsure
☐ Other Hispanic, Latino/a/x, or Spanish origin not listed (please describe):

☐ **Middle Eastern or North African**

If selected, are you:

☐ Egyptian
☐ Iranian
☐ Iraqi
☐ Israeli
☐ Lebanese
☐ Moroccan
☐ Syrian
☐ Unsure
☐ Other Middle Eastern or North African not listed:

☐ **Native Hawaiian or Other Pacific Islander**

If selected, are you:

☐ Native Hawaiian
☐ Chamorro
☐ Samoan
☐ Tongan
☐ Fijian
☐ Marshallese
☐ Unsure
☐ Other Pacific Islander not listed (please describe):

☐ **White, European American, or Caucasian**

If selected, are you:

☐ English
☐ French
☐ German
☐ Irish
☐ Italian
☐ Polish
☐ Scottish
☐ Unsure
☐ Other White not listed (please describe):

☐ **Something not named in list provided**

Please describe below:

My Intersecting Identities

☐ **Age and generational influences**

If selected, are you:

- ☐ Child
- ☐ Preteen
- ☐ Adolescent
- ☐ Emerging adult
- ☐ Middle aged
- ☐ Older adult
- ☐ Other age or generational category not listed:

☐ **Developmental or other disability**

If selected, are you:

- ☐ Cognitive
- ☐ Intellectual
- ☐ Sensory
- ☐ Physical
- ☐ Learning
- ☐ Mental health
- ☐ Other disability not listed (please describe):

☐ **Religion and spirituality**

If selected, are you:

- ☐ Buddhist
- ☐ Christian
- ☐ Hindu
- ☐ Jewish
- ☐ Muslim
- ☐ Spiritual (not religious)
- ☐ Unsure
- ☐ Other religion or spirituality not listed (please describe):

☐ **Socioeconomic status**

If selected, are you:

- ☐ Upper
- ☐ Middle
- ☐ Lower
- ☐ Unsure
- ☐ Other—I define my socioeconomic status as:

☐ **Sexual orientation**

If selected, are you:

- ☐ Asexual
- ☐ Bisexual
- ☐ Gay
- ☐ Heterosexual
- ☐ Lesbian
- ☐ Pansexual
- ☐ Queer
- ☐ Other sexual orientation not listed:

☐ **National origin**

If selected, are you:

- ☐ U.S.-born
- ☐ Immigrant
- ☐ Refugee
- ☐ International student
- ☐ Other national origin not listed (please describe):

☐ **Gender**

If selected, are you:

- ☐ Agender
- ☐ Female
- ☐ Male
- ☐ Nonbinary
- ☐ Transgender female
- ☐ Transgender male
- ☐ Unsure
- ☐ Gender not listed (please describe):

☐ **Something not named in list provided**

Please describe below:

Who Am I?

Fill out each box below with information collected in Chapter 1.

I am...	I like to do...
I can do...	I care about...

Who Am I?

Are there any **intersecting identities** that help you feel more connected with your racial and cultural background? If so, how do those intersecting identities influence your daily experiences as a POC?

Are there any intersecting identities that make it difficult to connect with your racial and cultural background? If so, how do those intersecting identities influence your daily experiences as a POC?

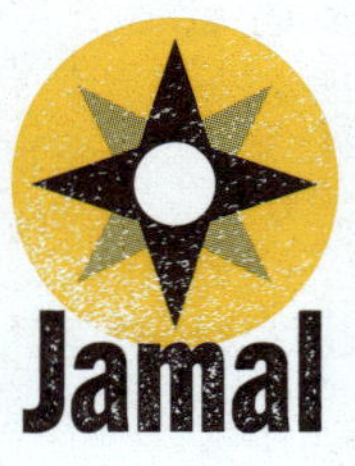

"I checked off being Black and Christian. But I added being a college graduate. That's an important part of how I see myself too."

"I CAN DO": WHAT ARE YOUR ABILITIES OR STRENGTHS?

Strengths describe any ability that *increases our chance of achieving our goals.* Think about your physical abilities (walking, running, jumping, dancing, balancing), your brain's abilities (solving problems, reading, writing), and your creative abilities (drawing, songwriting). Some strengths come naturally, and others require a lot of effort and practice to build up so they can help us pursue desired goals. What strengths do NOT mean for the purposes of this book is that your abilities have to reflect superhuman physical strength, an award-winning voice, or a pro-level jump shot to be considered a strength. Use the **My Strengths chart** on the next page to identify the abilities and traits you are able to (or want to learn to) use to help achieve your goals.

Fill In Your Who Am I? Diagram: Now write in the "I can do" square of the diagram on the facing page the personal strengths that you use most often in your daily life to achieve personal goals.

My Strengths

Abilities I currently use: *Circle (or check off)* the abilities and traits that you feel like you are able to use in your daily life to achieve important goals.

Abilities I want to develop: Place a *star/asterisk (or highlight)* beside the abilities and traits that you hope to grow to rely on them more frequently in daily life.

- ☐ Telling jokes
- ☐ Drawing
- ☐ Writing
- ☐ Running
- ☐ Balance/ coordination
- ☐ Easy-going
- ☐ Speak more than one language
- ☐ Dancing
- ☐ Curious
- ☐ Reading
- ☐ Caring
- ☐ Critical thinker
- ☐ Friendly
- ☐ Seeking support
- ☐ Kind
- ☐ Problem solver
- ☐ Math
- ☐ Giving
- ☐ Community builder
- ☐ Dependable
- ☐ Setting boundaries
- ☐ Good with money
- ☐ Organization
- ☐ Charming
- ☐ Independent
- ☐ Ambitious ("go getter")
- ☐ Teacher
- ☐ Patience
- ☐ Leader
- ☐ Nurturing
- ☐ Public speaking
- ☐ Creative
- ☐ Performing music
- ☐ Entrepreneur
- ☐ Resilience
- ☐ Trend setter
- ☐ Advocacy
- ☐ Historian
- ☐ Building relationships
- ☐ Effective communication
- ☐ Reading music
- ☐ Storytelling
- ☐ Video gaming
- ☐ Visual arts
- ☐ Soothing my emotions
- ☐ Listening
- ☐ Helping others soothe their emotions
- ☐ Being vulnerable
- ☐ Prayer
- ☐ Goal-oriented
- ☐ Hard working
- ☐ Being responsible
- ☐ Mindfulness
- ☐ Strategic
- ☐ Multi-tasking
- ☐ Knowledge of cultural traditions
- ☐ Flexible thinker
- ☐ Self-pride
- ☐ Fashionable
- ☐ Energetic
- ☐ Cares about environment
- ☐ Debating
- ☐ Trustworthy
- ☐ Other: ___________
- ☐ Other: ___________
- ☐ Other: ___________
- ☐ Other: ___________
- ☐ Other: ___________
- ☐ Other: ___________
- ☐ Other: ___________

Pause and Reflect on Your Personal Strengths

Society has a way of influencing which personal strengths POCs feel capable of having and even the abilities POCs feel expected to have. Take a few moments to reflect on how your strengths are connected with your racial and cultural background and record your thoughts below.

How did you learn that you possessed the abilities you selected?

Were any abilities learned or inspired by members of your racial and cultural community?

What does it feel like when you are in relationships or community spaces that allow you to use these strengths? Is it ever a source of pride to utilize these abilities?

Do you feel like any of the strengths you selected are connected with your racial and cultural background? If yes, how?

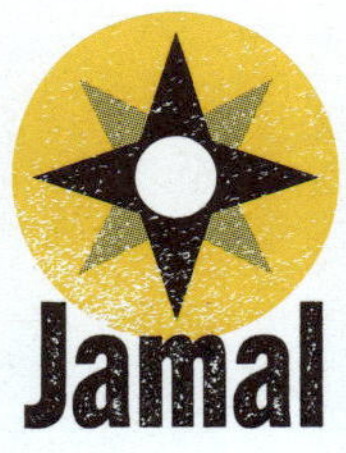

"Sometimes it's hard to remember what my strengths are. It was nice to think about the abilities I have and how they are connected to who I am."

"I LIKE TO DO": WHAT ARE YOUR INTERESTS?

Interests describe the types of activities that give us an opportunity to relax, experience joy or happiness, or feel accomplished. Have you ever considered whether you have any interests that are strongly connected with your racial and cultural background? Maybe you developed an interest through a tradition or custom associated with this part of your identity. Or you learned it from or participate in it with those in your racial and cultural community. Use the **My Interests chart** on the next page to identify what you like to do.

What about interests that don't fit what people expect from your racial and cultural background? If you've been expected to be into sports and hip-hop because you're Black, or to like spicy food and dancing because you're Latina, or to be most interested in math and science as an Asian American, you've been subjected to stereotyping. You may be a Black teen who prefers ballet, a Latina whose favorite

My Interests

1. My relaxing activities: List any activities you currently do to relax and recharge.

2. My fun activities: List any activities you currently do to have fun either when alone or with those closest to you.

3. My activities that make me feel accomplished: List any activities you currently do that help you feel accomplished or proud.

4. Activities I'd like to do: List any interests you have that you would like to spend more time doing.

food is Chinese and not Mexican, or an Asian American who loves to write and hates equations. In thinking of what you like to do, be sure to honor any preferred activities that are *your* interests instead of what others expect you to like.

Now Fill In Your Who Am I? Diagram: Write the interests you listed on page 18 in the square for "I like to do" on page 14.

Pause and Reflect on Your Interests

Personal interests are subjected to others' expectations just like personal strengths. When your interests naturally fit these expectations, it can feel great—like you belong and your interests are sincerely accepted. But when your surroundings do not fully support, understand, and embrace your interests, knowing when and where to invest time and energy into your interests may feel confusing. Take a few moments to reflect on the ways your interests do (or do not) fit into what is expected of someone with your racial and cultural background Write your thoughts below.

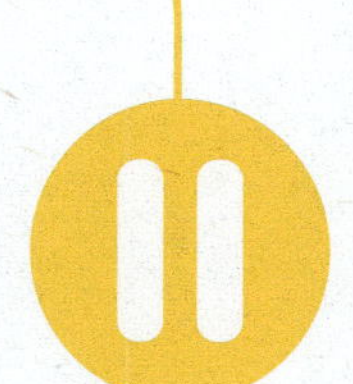

Which of your interests feel the most connected with your racial and cultural background—possibly because someone from your background introduced you to this interest or this interest is a way you celebrate being a member of your background?

How do your interests compare to what you think others expect you to be interested in?

How do your interests compare to those of other POCs that you typically interact with?

How does it feel to have these similarities with and differences from other POCs?

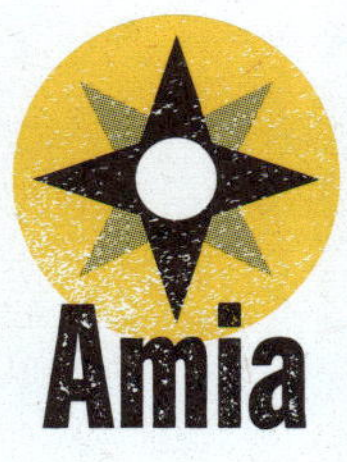

"I was able to use this part of the Who Am I? exercise to remember how much I enjoy singing and watching movies. I really want to get back to doing these activities."

"I CARE ABOUT": WHAT ARE YOUR VALUES?

Values describe any meaningful and important ideas, morals, or areas of life that we want to prioritize. A value is NOT a goal, but hopefully our values help us create our goals. Our values are often influenced by those who share our racial and cultural background. Over time, however, the values that people within our cultural community encourage us to embrace may become less and less personally meaningful to us. One way to learn about what we care most about in life is to complete the **Parts of My Life I Value Most diagram** on the facing page.

First, read through the examples of different parts of life that people may care a lot about.

Second, please use the scale below to rate how important you feel each area of life is to you right now and insert the number in the box below it. If you notice that

0 1 2 3 4 5 6 7 8 9 10
Not at all important to me
A little important to me
Somewhat important to me
Important to me
Very important to me

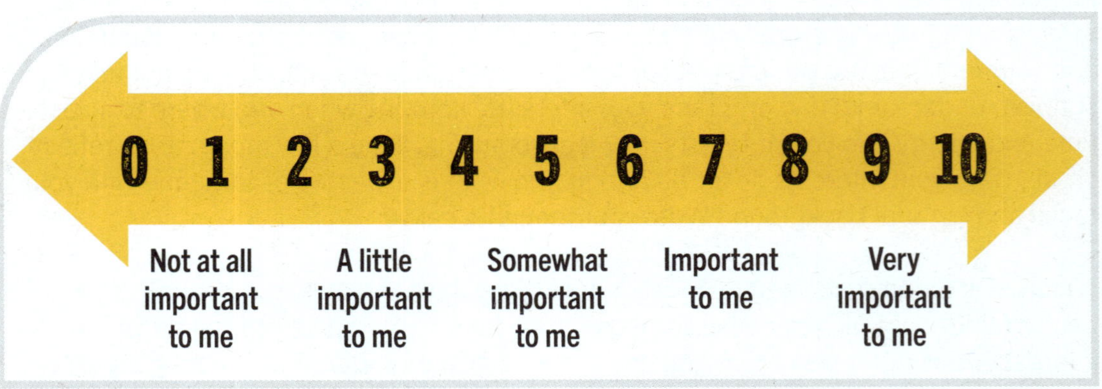

there are some areas of your life that are missing, please add them at the bottom of the diagram and rate how important they are to you.

Third, if you'd like to explore your specific values, read through the list below and *circle or highlight* any values that are important to you. You can find even more values by using the photo feature on your smartphone to scan either QR code after this list, on page 23.

Mindfulness. To pause and choose to be in the present moment.

Friendship. To be surrounded by supportive, understanding friends.

Nonconformity. To resist or not blindly follow authority and norms.

Family. To prioritize maintaining close connection with family.

Justice. To encourage fairness and equal treatment for all.

Mastery. To become able to skillfully complete important tasks and activities.

Challenge. To look for and attempt to complete hard tasks and problems.

Leisure. To create opportunities for relaxation, fun, and enjoyment.

Openness. To look for and invite new experiences in life.

Parts of My Life I Value Most

- My family relationships ☐
- My friendships ☐
- My romantic relationships ☐
- My peer/colleague relationships ☐
- My emotional well-being ☐
- My physical well-being ☐
- My spiritual well-being ☐
- My community's well-being ☐
- My job/career (current or future) ☐
- My education ☐
- My hobbies/fun activities ☐
- My personal growth ☐

Other (insert any areas of life that you also care about):

Independence. To provide for needs and wants without depending on others.

Cooperation. To team up and work well with others.

Helpfulness. To be supportive to others.

Cultural harmony. To participate in cultural practices and uphold cultural values.

Growth. To search for and be open to change and improvement.

God's will. To look for and align life with God's will.

Self-acceptance. To embrace and love self just as it is.

Health and fitness. To prioritize activities that promote emotional and physical wellness.

Loving. To offer care and compassion to others.

Self-control. To be intentional with and in control of my actions.

Creativity. To explore, produce, and showcase new ideas.

Passion. To have strong feelings and opinions about self and the surrounding world.

Faithfulness. To be reliable and trustworthy within relationships.

Contribution. To have a meaningful, lasting impact on the world.

Tradition. To align life with customs and beliefs that have been passed down.

Wealth. To possess a lot of money.

Hardworking. To work hard and well at life tasks.

Service. To tend to another's needs and wants.

Popularity. To be liked and admired by a lot of people.

Flexibility. To be able to easily adapt to new experiences.

Genuineness. To carry self and make decisions in ways that accurately represent self.

Simplicity. To lead a simple lifestyle with few needs or wants.

Generosity. To search for opportunities to offer possessions or resources to others.

Humor. To look for chances to laugh and make jokes.

Beauty. To pause and enjoy the beauty in surroundings.

Intimacy. To be vulnerable and share important details about self with others.

List any additional values that are important to you below:

___

___

___

Now Fill In Your Who Am I? Diagram: Write the parts of life or specific values that are most important to you in the square for "I care about" on page 14.

Pause and Reflect on Your Values

Our values are greatly impacted by our relationships and the community spaces where we spend most of our time. Take a moment and think about how your values are connected to your racial and cultural background and write in your thoughts below.

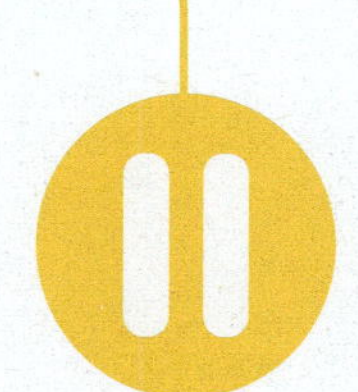

Who are the people who have had the greatest influences on what you care about the most right now in your life? Are any of these people members of your racial and cultural background?

Are any of your values connected with how you try to express your racial and cultural background?

Which of your values seem most and least supported by others who share your racial and cultural background?

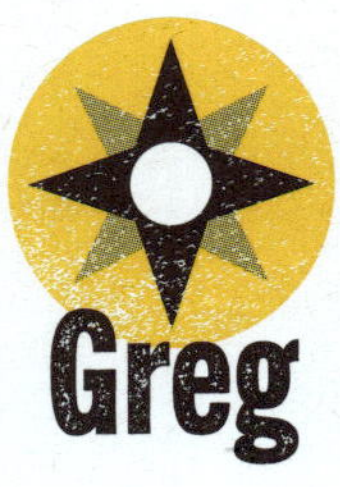

"I really care about my education and my family. I really want to make sure my decisions honor these areas of my life."

Chapter 1: Recap and Reflect

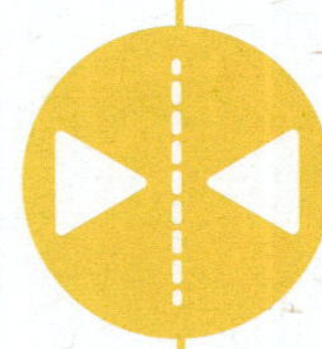

RECAP

- In this workbook, **persons of color (POCs)** refers to people whose racial and cultural backgrounds cause them to have certain shared experiences that include facing culturally stressful events.
- **Racial background** refers to the ways people are labeled or categorized based on their physical characteristics.
- **Cultural background** refers to the customs, traditions, interests, languages, and general daily experiences that are unique to POCs.
- The **Who Am I? diagram** is a tool that helps us understand the parts of ourselves that are most important to us.

REFLECT

Give yourself a pat on the back for taking the time to think carefully about yourself through the pausing and reflecting exercises in this chapter. Now take a few more moments to think about your reactions to your completed Who Am I? diagram.

What parts of your Who Am I? diagram help you feel most connected to your racial and cultural background?

What parts of your Who Am I? diagram do you feel most proud of?

Are there any parts of your Who Am I? diagram that have caused you to feel unfairly judged, mistreated, or denied opportunities? If so, which parts?

2 Have I Experienced Cultural Stress?

Chapter 1 helped you explore who you are, particularly in the context of your racial and cultural background. It's unfortunate that not everyone appreciates the rich cultural experiences that POCs have. The hurtful beliefs and attitudes that categorize some groups as inferior have given rise to culturally stressful events in the daily lives of POCs for generations. As shown in the diagram below, these events can be caused by relationship and community stressors that have already arisen, are

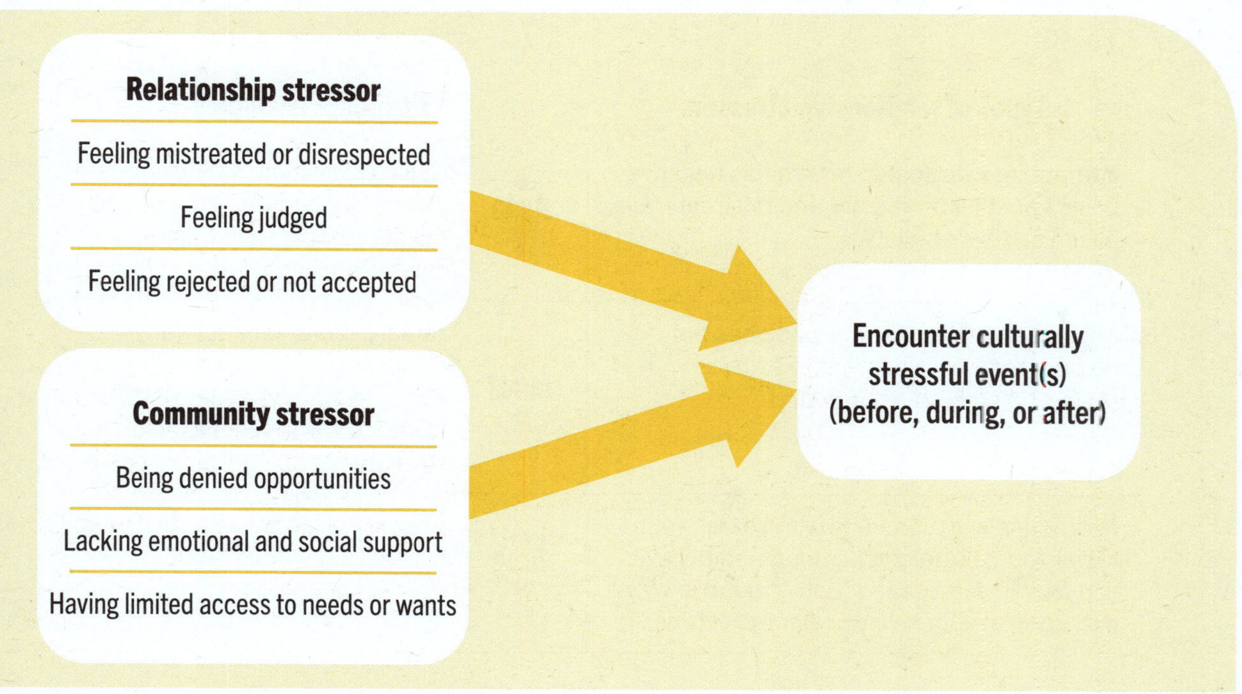

arising right now, or could arise in the future. In this chapter, you will learn which relationships and community spaces have been your greatest sources of cultural stress.

WHAT IS A RELATIONSHIP STRESSOR?

A **relationship stressor** is often at work when we feel that someone else's beliefs and attitudes about our racial and cultural backgrounds create a complicated, uncomfortable, or even confrontational social interaction. Such beliefs and attitudes can include viewing POCs as dangerous and criminal or considering POCs to lack intelligence and capable skill sets. They can also include treating POCs as outsiders who do not belong or behaving as if their cultural traditions and perspectives are not important or credible. It's important to note, however, that relationship stressors can be created in interactions between POCs, including with family and friends, not just between POCs and non-POC individuals.

When racially and culturally biased beliefs and attitudes reveal themselves in social interactions, they can trigger uncomfortable emotions, leave us unsure what to say or do, and even impact how we think or feel about ourselves. It's important to cope with such stressors. But, knowing how to cope can be hard if we don't notice this source of cultural stress when it's happening. It can help to think of relationship stressors as falling into three categories, as shown in the table below.

Types of relationship stressors	Navigator examples	
Interacting with someone who has negative beliefs about who you are and mistreats you based on these beliefs	Amia	Amia's classmate makes an insensitive comment about her religious background during a class discussion.
Interacting with someone who does not respect the ways you want to express your racial and cultural background	Jamal	Jamal's coworkers appear disinterested in the topics he wants to discuss and instead want to interact with him based on their stereotypes about Black people.
Interacting with someone who shares your racial and cultural background and believes you should express that background in ways that conflict with how you want to express it	Greg	Greg is teased by other POCs for his musical interests and academic ambitions.

All our navigators have been subjected to the three types of relationship stress.

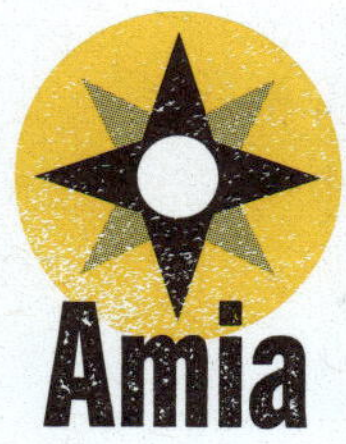

One day Amia's classmate Rick singled her out when expressing his negative beliefs and feelings about her Islamic faith in the middle of class. Worse, after class he approached her and had the audacity to accuse Amia of being "too sensitive" when she became tearful upon hearing him repeat his negative beliefs to her while they were alone. Being confronted with someone's negativity about our racial and cultural background can be emotionally triggering and create a sense of urgency to respond: *"Do I call out their ignorance and try to educate? "Do I show them with my actions how inaccurate their beliefs are?" "Do I ignore their ignorance and try to move on with my life?"*

Pause and Reflect on Amia's Relationship Stressor

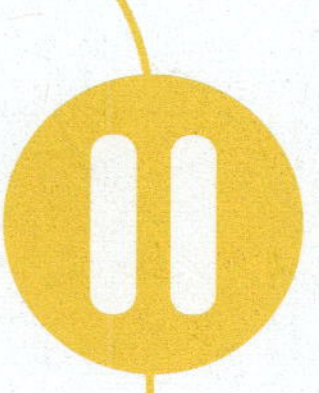

Rick's decision to express his negative beliefs forced Amia to make a decision about how to respond in the moment but left her feeling blindsided and confused about what to do. Can you relate to how Amia felt while talking to Rick? If so, take a moment to describe below:

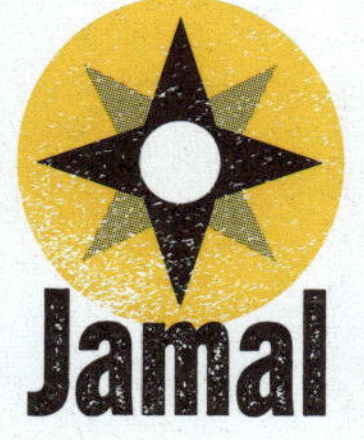

At an after-work event, Jamal tried to connect with his colleagues by simply being himself and showcasing different parts of his Who Am I? diagram. For context, his diagram includes his:

- Identities: Being Black, Christian, male, and a college graduate
- Strengths: Good with numbers, people person, and creative
- Interests: Anime, reality television, and cooking
- Values: Family, friendship, and achievement

And, when Jamal tried to share these parts of himself at the event, none of his coworkers showed any interest, which left him wanting to get out of there as soon as possible.

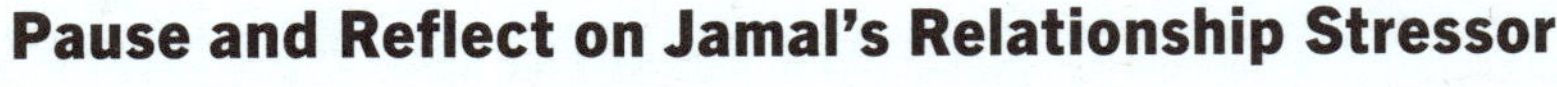

Pause and Reflect on Jamal's Relationship Stressor

Can you relate to Jamal's feeling as if his true self was not seen as worth being acknowledged or celebrated by his colleagues? Such a lack of acceptance or feelings of rejection can also happen within friendships, among family, or when meeting new people. If you can relate, take a moment to describe below:

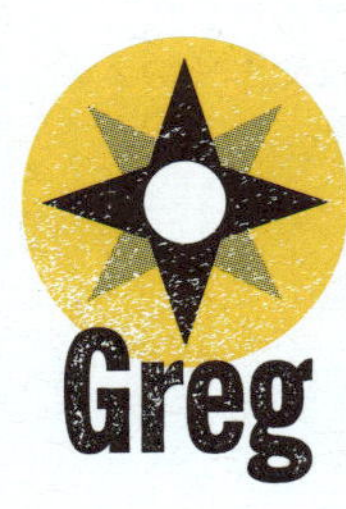

Greg has big dreams for his future and is really excited to pursue them. But he's been repeatedly teased and criticized by his Latino and Black peers for expressing the parts of himself that are connected with these dreams—often being judged as "acting White" or not being Latino enough. Though our family, friends, and members of our racial and cultural group can be an amazingly useful resource, feeling judged and not accepted by those who share our backgrounds can be emotionally stressful and make it hard to develop love and appreciation for who we are.

Pause and Reflect on Greg's Relationship Stressor

Have you ever had people within your racial and cultural background disagree with your dating choices or how you choose to observe religious practices, judge your knowledge and use of your native language, or generally disapprove of how you observe any cultural tradition? If so, take a moment to describe below:

WHAT IS A COMMUNITY STRESSOR?

Our communities consist of spaces where we hang out, the resources offered within these spaces, and the laws and policies that govern how residents navigate these spaces. For POCs, **community stressors** describe moments when different community spaces, such as schools, jobs, housing developments, or even health care clinics, lack the supports and protection they need. Unfortunately, our society continues to be impacted by *systemic racism*, which can be defined as the ways laws, policies, and communitywide decisions create unequal opportunity for many POCs. These roots of racism have impacted communities for decades and become so deeply woven into the natural rhythms of everyday life that they often escape notice. To help you pause and notice the possible effects of systemic racism on your daily experiences, think of community stressors as falling into three categories, shown in the following table.

Examples of community stressors	Navigator examples
Being in an environment that generally lacks resources for you to pursue important goals	Greg: Greg is raised in a community that does not offer a sense of safety, educational opportunity, or financial stability—all resources that he feels would support his ability to achieve his academic goals.
Being in an environment that lacks racial and cultural diversity	Jamal: Jamal is one of only a few POCs at his job, which makes it hard for him to feel supported or feel as if he has equal opportunity to excel in his workplace.
Being in an environment that feels unsupportive and lacks protection	Amia: Amia does not feel as if her classroom and more broadly her school offer her support and protection from ongoing culturally stressful experiences.

Again, our navigators have experienced all three types of community stress.

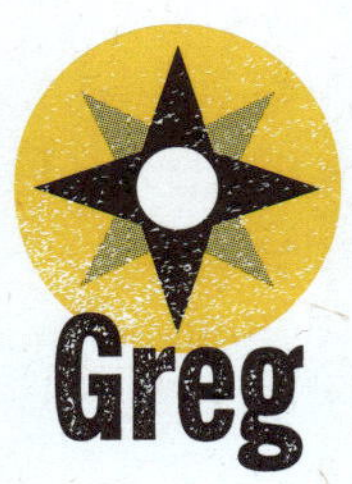

Many years ago Greg's community was considered an "industrial city" because most of its residents worked at the local factory. At that time, most of its residents were White—until Black and Latino Americans began moving in, which spurred a White flight. Unfortunately, about 10 years ago, the owners of the local factory felt Greg's community was no longer a good fit for their company and shut down the factory—effectively eliminating the biggest employer in their community. Today, Greg's community is plagued by poverty and does not offer him access to the career opportunities that would encourage him to remain there. To an extent, systemic racism in Greg's community also reduces his access to good-quality education, health care, affordable housing, and healthy food options.

Pause and Reflect on Greg's Community Stressor

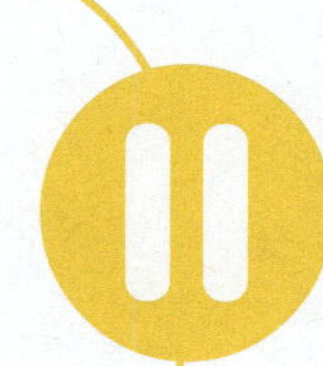

Are there any opportunities or resources that you wish your neighborhood, school, job, or broader community offered you? If so, take a moment to describe below:

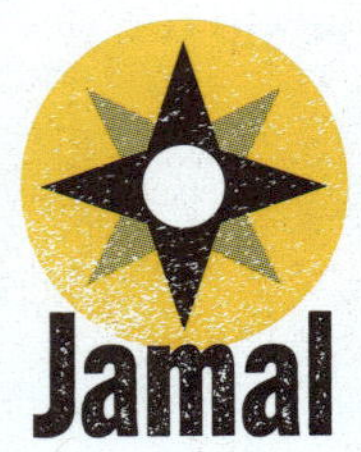

Jamal's academic success has granted him an opportunity to enter corporate America. So far, the absence of racial and cultural diversity throughout his academic journey and now at work has created obstacles that Jamal has had to learn to navigate. He doesn't have the sense of belonging and connection that would support his ability to grow in his job, and he doesn't have the outlet of relaxing after work with colleagues who see and get him. Instead, he often feels exhausted by having to mask certain parts of himself and works hard daily to be accepted by his colleagues and bosses. Jamal isn't sure who to trust at work and hasn't found a mentor who could help him navigate this space and develop his career.

Pause and Reflect on Jamal's Community Stressor

Have you ever found yourself in social spaces where you were the only one from your racial and cultural background? Or possibly have you noticed that you struggle to know who in your surroundings you can trust to offer you support and guidance? If so, take a moment to describe below:

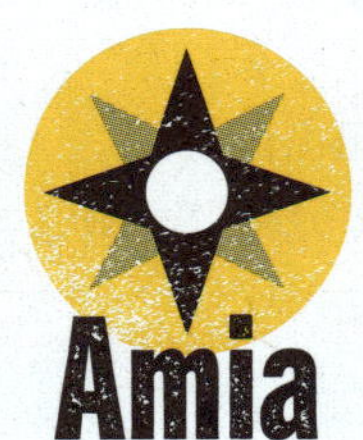

Amia's interactions with judgmental peers like Rick create for her an urgent need for *relational* and *systemic* support at school and elsewhere. Yet when Rick openly expressed negative beliefs about her racial and cultural background, his remarks were met with silence from her teacher and other classmates. Amia needed a support network or allies within the school that she could go to whenever she had concerns or needs, but her school provided neither relational nor systemic aid—no friends spoke up on her behalf and no punitive or corrective actions from the teacher addressed her classmate's insensitive behavior.

Pause and Reflect on Amia's Community Stressor

Can you relate to Amia's feeling unsupported and unprotected at her school? Or maybe you've wished that people within your surroundings, such as friends, family, teacher, coworkers, or bosses, would take action and help stop culturally stressful events from happening. If so, take a moment to describe below:

HOW TO CREATE A RELATIONSHIP AND COMMUNITY MAP

Now that you have a better sense of what relationship and community stressors can look like, you're ready to get a snapshot of any cultural stressors in your surroundings. The relationship and community map shown here gives you a place to identify the people you are surrounded by and the places in your community where you spend time. The concentric circles give you a way to see how close the people you interact with are to you and where you spend most of your time in your community. Start by reading the navigator's relationship and community map. Then you'll have a chance to fill in your own map.

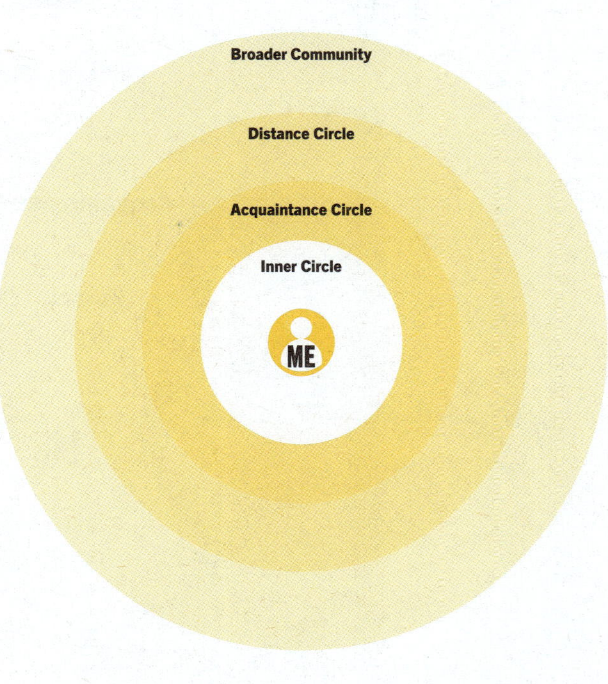

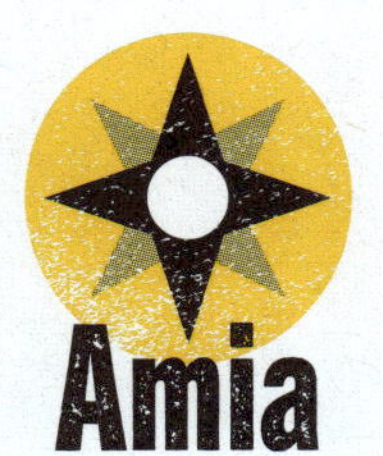

Amia's Relationship and Community Map

As Amia discovered, filling out a Relationship and Community Map can be an eye opener. Looking at Amia's map on the next page, you can see that she feels most connected with her mother, cousin, middle sister, English as Second Language (ESL) teacher, and her close friends at her mosque—those in her inner circle. Amia does not feel as close with her father because they tend not to see eye to eye on how she should carry herself as a Muslim woman. She also has a somewhat good relationship with two POC classmates and a youth leader at her mosque—they all make Amia feel comfortable to chat with, but she definitely does not discuss anything too deep or vulnerable. They all fit into Amia's acquaintance circle. We can also see that Amia's experiences with two White classmates, Thomas and Rick, have not only landed them in the distanced circle, but that Amia has become uncomfortable interacting with most of her White-presenting classmates. Due to some of her experiences since immigrating to the United States, she struggles to trust White-presenting people. And it seems that her history teacher's silence in response to Rick's comments has left her feeling unsure of him as well. Finally, the broader community circle of her map shows where in her community she spends most of her time.

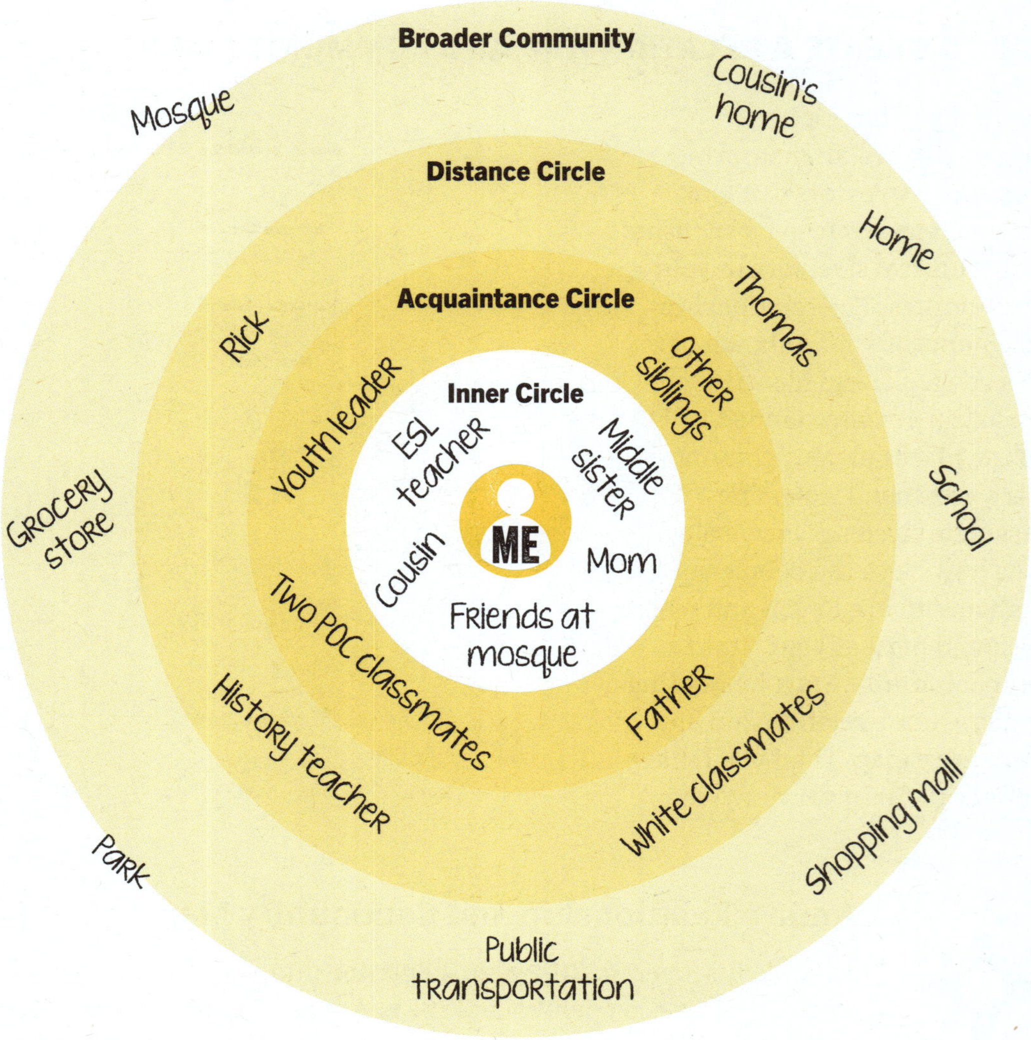

Broader Community

Mosque

Cousin's home

Home

School

Shopping mall

Public transportation

Park

Grocery store

Distance Circle

Rick

Thomas

White classmates

History teacher

Acquaintance Circle

Youth leader

Other siblings

Father

Two POC classmates

Inner Circle

ESL teacher

Middle sister

Mom

Friends at mosque

Cousin

ME

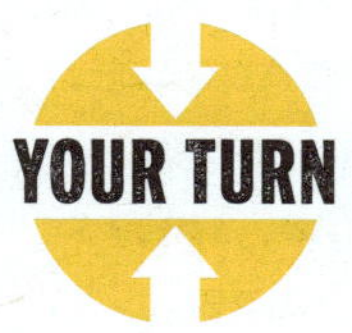

It's important to take time to fill in your relationship and community map (page 33), as you will use this map thoughtfully to help identify where you are most impacted by the types of relationship and community stressors imposing on Jamal, Greg, and Amia.

1. Fill in your inner circle. Enter the names of people in your life who offer you the most emotional and social support. These are the people you trust the most and are willing to be your most authentic self around. Such people can include parents/caregivers, close relatives, close friends (BFFs), mentors, coaches, or a therapist.

My Relationship and Community Map

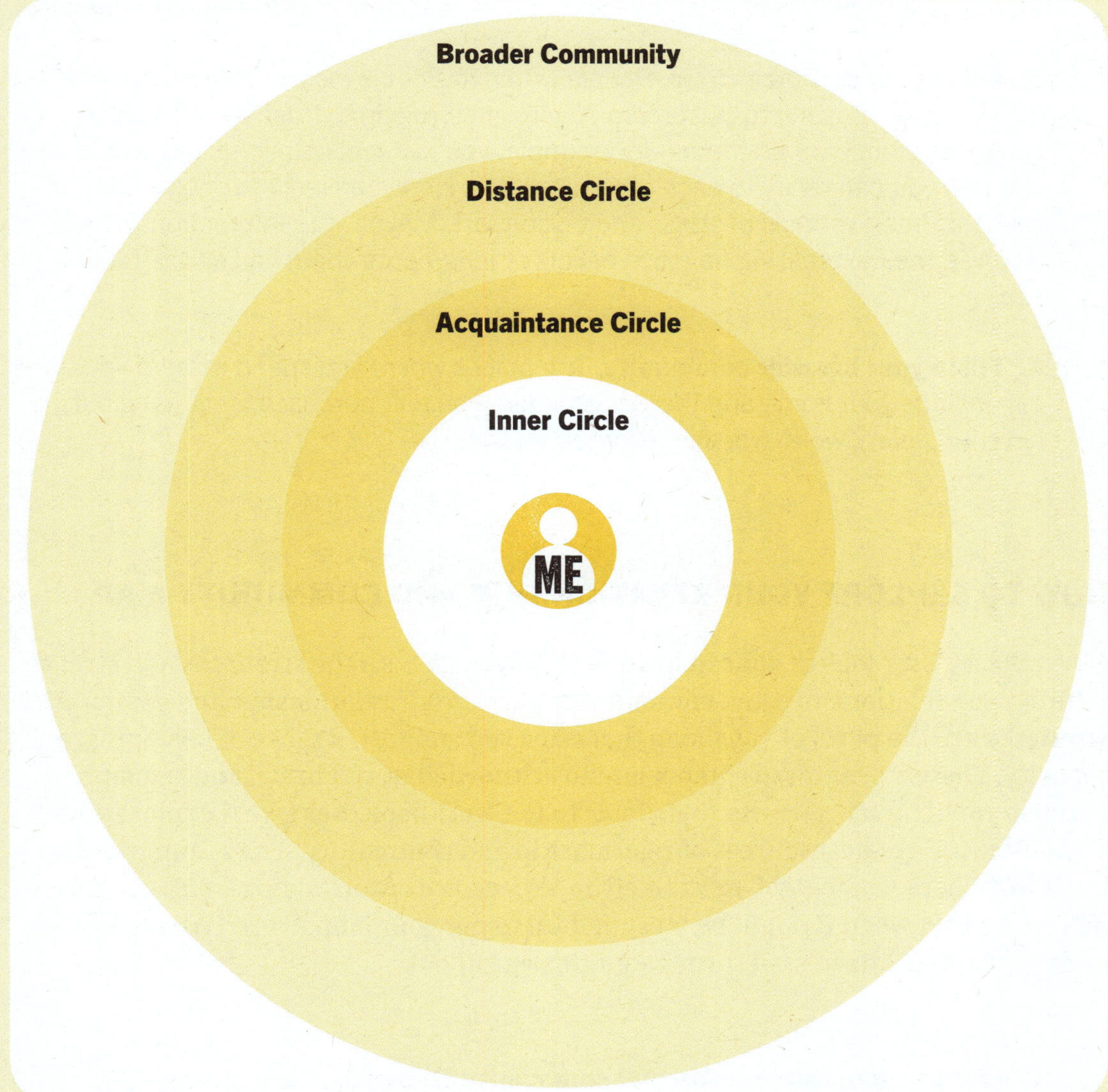

2. Fill in your acquaintance circle. Write in the names of people you are familiar with but with whom you find yourself remaining a bit guarded. You can connect with the people in this circle on specific topics or interests. Or you have shared experiences within a specific area of your life, but you wouldn't call them close friends. These people can include classmates, teachers, coworkers, or teammates.

3. Fill in your distance circle. People within this circle include those who have given you reasons not to trust them. You might struggle to trust them because you're less familiar with them—for example, you just met someone and aren't sure whether you can relate to each other. Also, this circle can include people who have primarily been sources of stress and discomfort. Maybe your interactions have involved their expressing negative beliefs or judgments about you or mistreating you.

4. Fill in your broader community. The places where you spend most of your time can include your home and the places where you eat, purchase food, hang out, have fun, learn, work, worship, exercise, or travel.

HOW TO EXPLORE YOUR RELATIONSHIP AND COMMUNITY MAP

Now take a closer look at your map and acknowledge both the strengths and stresses within your relationships and community spaces. Your relationship and community strengths are the parts of your map that offer you support, a sense of belonging, and security. These strengths are important to acknowledge, celebrate, and remember because you'll be asked to use them later in the workbook. Next we'll explore where you notice the greatest sources of relationship and community stress. Importantly, knowing where you feel the most likely to experience culturally stressful events will help you know when it might be most helpful to put your empowered coping hat on and use the skills discussed throughout this workbook.

1. Identify your relationship and community strengths. Most people don't achieve their goals or cope with life's obstacles without the support of people around them or without depending on parts of their community. Our relationships and community spaces can grant us access to the resources listed in the **My Social Resources lists** on the facing page. Under each heading are prompts that will help you explore whether any person or place within your map offers you each resource.

Using the lists on page 35, *circle or highlight* the people or places on your filled-in Relationship and Community Map (page 33) that offer you any of the

My Social Resources

Emotional Support (ES)

Are there any relationships or parts of your community that:

- Helps you feel safe to express your emotions
- Seeks to understand and listen to your emotions
- Helps you cope with your emotions in a healthy way

Social Support (SS)

Are there any relationships or parts of your community that:

- Praises your successes
- Shares similar lived experiences
- Gives you guidance on how to achieve your goals

Confident Self-Expression (CSE)

Are there any relationships or parts of your community that:

- Helps you feel safe to express yourself
- Allows you to celebrate your racial and cultural background
- Helps you explore what you love and appreciate about your background

Financial Stability (FS)

Are there any relationships or parts of your community that:

- Supports your ability to afford the things you "need" and "want"
- Helps you to reduce any worry about your ability to afford things now (or in the future)
- Helps you to feel confident you can pursue future financial goals

Sense of Safety (SOS)

Are there any relationships or parts of your community that:

- Helps you feel safe to hang out or walk around within your community
- Helps you know where danger is (or is not) within your community
- Helps you know what to do or how to protect yourself from danger within your community

New Ideas/Opportunities (NI/O)

Are there any relationships or parts of your community that:

- Exposes you to different types of activities and experiences
- Exposes you to different types of cultural groups
- Challenges you to think in new ways

six resources. You may find it helpful to use different-colored markers, crayons, colored pencils, or pens to color-code your map. Doing so can help you more easily see which resources you have the most access to on your map. For example: red = emotional support; blue = social support; orange = confident self-expression; green = financial stability; yellow = sense of safety; gray = new ideas/opportunities.

2. **Identify relationship stressors you've experienced.** Earlier in this chapter, our navigators showed three ways that a relationship stressor can occur. The diagram on the facing page lists statements or types of interactions that can cause such stress. This list can help you enhance your ability to recognize relationship stress. Carefully review these examples and place a check beside any you've experienced. (There are also spaces at the bottom to add any other relationship stressors you've experienced.)

3. **Identify the sources of relationship stress on your map.** Now that you've identified examples of relationship stressors you've experienced, put an X beside each person you feel has interacted with you or will interact with you in these ways. Remember, a relationship stressor can occur in interactions with both non-POCs and POCs.

4. **Identify community stressors you've experienced.** Earlier in the chapter, our navigators showed three ways that community stress can occur. As with relationship stressors, you can enhance your ability to notice community stressors by reviewing, in the diagram on page 38, the examples of how community spaces can lack the resources and supports that we need to thrive and achieve. Carefully review these examples and place a check beside any that feel like a community stressor you have experienced. Also, at the bottom, there are spaces for you to add any other community stressors you've experienced.

5. **Identify the sources of community stress on your map.** Finally, put an X beside each community space that you feel has or will be a community stressor.

My Relationship Stressors

"I don't think those people are that smart."

"This is America. We speak English here."

"You are so exotic looking. What are you?"

"You should go back to where you came from."

"Your hair does not look professional."

"Are you really sure that you can get into that school?"

"Immigrants ruined the economy."

"You are so articulate. I didn't expect that from you."

"You can't sit here."

"Aren't you supposed to be good at sports?"

"Lighter skin is just prettier to me. Is that wrong of me to say?"

Store clerk follows you around the store.

"Stop acting so White."

You are told, "You have to toughen up" after experiencing a culturally stressful event.

"People like us can't make mistakes. You have to be perfect."

"I hear an accent . . . Where are your people from?"

"You are not honoring or respecting us."

"Why do you wear that?"

"How did someone like you get such a job?"

"Are you sure they weren't just joking," after reporting an incident of cultural stress.

Add your example:

Add your example:

Add your example:

Add your example:

My Community Stressors

Noticing laws or policies are not equally and fairly enforced for people who look like you

"I am qualified, but I didn't get an interview."

Not having translation services available when needed

"I worked so hard and I don't understand why I wasn't picked."

Feeling as if you (and your family) do not have the financial resources you want or need

Walking into spaces and not seeing anyone who looks like you

Difficulty accessing educational supports needed

Feeling unsafe walking through your neighborhood

Not having access to teachers/mentors that share your racial/cultural background

"No matter how hard I try, others keep getting selected and I don't."

"I don't get the luxury to forget that I am a person of color ... I am reminded everywhere I go."

"My cultural experiences are not represented in the books I have to read."

Lacking opportunities to engage in your cultural traditions or practices

Noticing that your school doesn't have the resources you need to achieve your academic goals

Not having people stand up for you or against cultural stress

Unable to find health providers that share your racial/cultural background

Lacking opportunities to pursue the goals you have for yourself

Add your example:

Add your example:

Add your example:

Add your example:

Chapter 2: Recap and Reflect

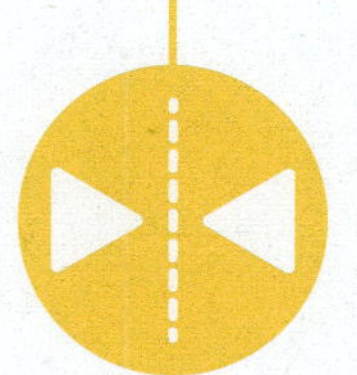

RECAP

- **Relationship stressors** and **community stressors** are what cause us to experience culturally stressful events.
- **Relationship stressors** arise when we feel the people around us have or might negatively judge, disrespect, or mistreat us due to our racial and cultural background.
- **Community stressors** arise when different community spaces cause us to feel unsupported or unprotected.
- Your **Relationship and Community Map** is a way to represent both the strengths and stresses within your surroundings.

REFLECT

Congrats! You have done some great work identifying the strengths and sources of cultural stress in your surroundings. Take a few moments to reflect on the following prompts and write in your responses. Doing so will help you complete the exercise in the next chapter.

Which **relationships** and **community spaces** make you feel least likely to experience culturally stressful events?

Which **relationships** and **community spaces** offer you the most support when you experience a culturally stressful event?

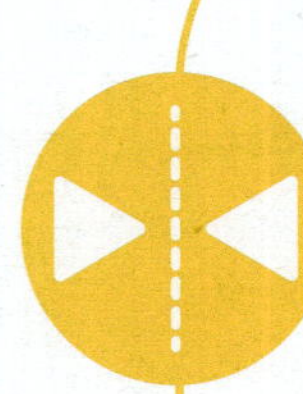

If you've experienced **relationship stressors** within your inner circles, how does it feel to experience such cultural stress from people in your inner circle compared to people in other circles?

Which **community stressors** feel most impactful to your day-to-day experiences?

3 How Have I Been Impacted by Cultural Stress?

Whenever you notice a culturally stressful event, it's important to understand how it impacted you right then and how it might continue to do so. This knowledge equips you to select the best coping skills for healing in that moment and for navigating future stressful events. This chapter introduces three broad ways that cultural stress may affect you and then helps you clarify which you are most interested in learning to cope with by completing a brief questionnaire.

WHAT ARE THE IMPACTS OF CULTURAL STRESS?

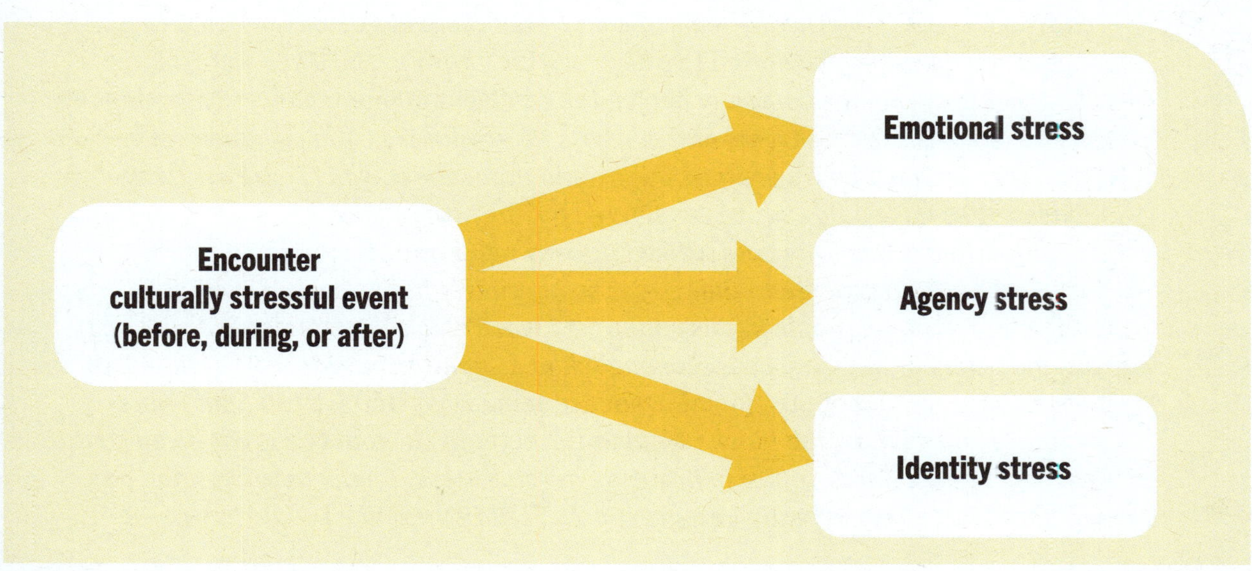

Culturally stressful events can affect our emotions, our sense of agency and control, and how we think and feel about the racial and cultural aspects of our identity. Cultural stress can result from one major event, like witnessing a person from your community being assaulted by a police officer. Or it can result from seemingly small, everyday interactions with the people around us.

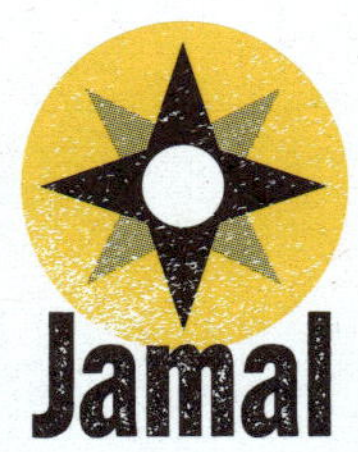

Jamal gave this account of a particularly stressful day he had at work.

It was a typical Monday morning with the same routine—30 minutes of exercise, quick bite of breakfast, and then off to work. Today I made it out of the apartment on time—the day was off to a good start. While walking to the office, I came up alongside a group of women who kept glancing in my direction. At first I was like "Maybe they think I'm cute!" But then they did something odd—they looked at me, looked at each other, crossed the street, and then kept walking in the same direction as me. Weird, right? But I eventually forgot about them and kept it moving.

Before I knew it, I was at work and went straight into a team meeting. During this meeting, my boss decided to comment on a recent act of police brutality directed at a Black man in our community that has been all over the news. He asked us all to reflect openly about how such events make us feel. I immediately became annoyed—like why do I have to sit here and listen to all my White colleagues debate about whether police brutality is even a real thing? Ugh, I don't get paid enough for this. I managed to get through the meeting without saying anything, but, wow, I have some ignorant colleagues.

The day moved on as a typical Monday does. But, while taking a quick bathroom break, I overheard some of my White colleagues discussing that they applied for the same promotion I've been working hard to get. They were joking about being new to the company but feeling confident in their chances of getting the position because their parents and our boss all graduated from the same college. From then on, my day was ruined. All I could think about was "There's no way someone like me would ever be considered for the promotion."

A few hours later, my boss walked into my office and started saying, "Hey, Jamal, what the police did to that guy is so horrible. I feel so sorry for what is happening to Black people in this country." I wasn't sure how to respond, so I just sat and listened. Next, my boss seemingly had a spontaneous idea: "We should do something about all of this. Jamal, what are some ways that we can fight police brutality and support the Black community? Actually, it would be great if you could lead a committee in the office to brainstorm some ideas. I unfortunately can't pay you for it, but it would really be a great help." I didn't feel like I could say no—I mean I want the promotion, right? So, I answered, "Sure, why not?" Fortunately, my workday ended soon after that. I made my way home, and as soon as I got into the house, I plopped down onto the couch, thinking, "Man, today was exhausting and it's only Monday."

Jamal has his eyes set on that promotion. He's working hard and feels like he's making meaningful steps toward that goal. But the stress kept piling on him today, from the awkward interaction with the women on the sidewalk to hearing his White colleagues debate about police brutality to feeling disadvantaged in the competition for the promotion to being tagged to lead his company's activism efforts. These experiences can be used to illustrate three ways cultural stress can impact your life, as shown in the following table.

Cultural Stress During Jamal's Workday

Type of cultural stress impact	Definition	Coping challenges
Emotional stress	Strong and hurtful emotions felt in response to culturally stressful events. Such emotions can include anger, anxiety, sadness, numbness.	Jamal felt annoyed, hopeless, and ultimately exhausted by these work experiences.
Agency stress	Feeling a lack of control and feeling unsure what to say or do to endure, stop, or limit exposure to culturally stressful events.	When asked to take lead on a committee focused on police brutality, Jamal did not feel he could say no to his boss.
Identity stress	Struggling to develop and maintain self-love, self-confidence, or cultural pride when exposed to culturally stressful events.	After learning about the academic connection his White colleagues had with their boss, Jamal thought, "There's no way someone like me would ever be considered [for the promotion]."

Jamal's experiences in his workday causing him to undergo emotional, agency, and identity stresses are unfortunately not uncommon. It's rare for a culturally stressful event to have only one of the three stressful impacts. Knowing which ones have affected you in a certain situation can help you choose the best skill sets to use to make empowered coping decisions, as you'll see later in this book.

Pause and Reflect on Your Cultural Stress Impacts

Before moving ahead in the chapter, complete the questionnaire on pages 45–46. Doing so will help you start exploring the impacts of cultural stress on your life and help you set goals for using the rest of this book.

YOUR WORKBOOK GOALS

Thank you for taking the time to fill out the questionnaire. The final step before launching into this journey of growing your empowered coping abilities is to clarify what you hope to get out of completing this book. Before you do, here's a summary of what's to come:

Part Two: Emotional stress	Learning how to notice what your emotional stress looks and feels like Learning coping decisions for managing your emotional stress in ways that you are proud of
Part Three: Agency stress	Learning how to notice when you are being impacted by agency stress Learning coping decisions that can help you stand up for yourself and meaningfully remain within these relationships and parts of your community (when needed)
Part Four: Identity stress	Learning how to notice when you are struggling to maintain self-love, self-confidence, and cultural pride Learning coping decisions that can help you grow and protect your self-love, self-confidence, and cultural pride
Part Five: Putting it all together	Learning how to identify all the ways a specific culturally stressful event may be impacting you in real time Learning how to choose the coping decisions that are best for the moment you are in

Now that you have a general sense of what to expect, use the questions in the worksheet on page 47 to state your goals for completing the workbook. Use your questionnaire responses to help you decide which parts of the book feel the most important to you. Also, you may find it helpful to discuss your questionnaire responses with one of your own navigators (the people you listed on page 6). Such support may help you more clearly state your goals for the workbook or discover goals that you had not considered before.

Cultural Stress Impact Questionnaire

1. **List culturally stressful events.** Looking back at your Relationship and Community Map (page 33), list below any past, present, or anticipated culturally stressful events that you've experienced (or may experience) while interacting with the people and community spaces on your map.

Culturally Stressful Events in My Relationships and Community

2. **Assess the emotional stress impact.** We can feel various strong and hurtful emotions when we've been judged, mistreated, or denied an opportunity because of some part of our identity. Unfortunately, it can be hard to recognize these emotions at the time or know what to do when feeling them. Below, please describe any signs of *emotional stress* you've experienced in response to the culturally stressful events you listed in step 1.

My Emotional Stress in Response to Culturally Stressful Events

What types of emotions have you felt in response to the culturally stressful events you listed above? *Examples can include anxiety, fear, anger, rage, sadness, depression, numbness, confusion.*	
Have you ever felt *unable to name or describe your emotions* in response to these events?	o Yes o No o Not sure
Have you ever *become critical or judgmental of your emotions* after experiencing these events?	o Yes o No o Not sure
Have you ever *felt unsure of how to cope* with your emotions in response to these events?	o Yes o No o Not sure
Are there any other ways that a culturally stressful event has impacted you emotionally?	o Yes o No o Not sure
If yes, please describe:	

(continued)

Cultural Stress Impact Questionnaire *(page 2 of 2)*

3. **Assess the agency stress impact.** Feeling a lack of agency or control when faced with culturally stressful events can take shape as feeling unsure what to say or do to endure, stop, or limit exposure to these experiences. Below, please describe any signs of *agency stress* you have experienced in response to the culturally stressful events you listed.

My Agency Stress in Response to Culturally Stressful Events in My Relationships and Community

Have you ever felt unsure how to confront or address a *person (or group of people)* who you felt was mistreating, judging, or denying you an opportunity due to your race or cultural background?	o Yes o No o Not sure
Have you ever wanted to change or improve a *community space* that felt unsupportive, unsafe, or unfair, but felt unsure how to do so?	o Yes o No o Not sure
Are there any other ways that a culturally stressful event has impacted your sense of agency and control?	o Yes o No o Not sure
If yes, please describe:	

4. **Assess the identity stress impact.** Feeling stress about who you are involves struggling to experience self-love, self-confidence, and overall cultural pride due to culturally stressful events. Below, please describe any signs of *identity stress* you've experienced in response to the culturally stressful events you listed.

My Identity Stress in Response to Culturally Stressful Events in My Relationships and Community

Have you ever had moments when you struggled to feel positive about any part of your racial and cultural background?	o **Yes** o **No** o **Not sure**
Have you ever wanted to learn more about your racial and cultural background, but felt unsure how to go about exploring this part of yourself?	o **Yes** o **No** o **Not sure**
Have you ever struggled to confidently express parts of your racial and cultural background within any relationships or community spaces?	o **Yes** o **No** o **Not sure**
Are there any other ways that a culturally stressful event has impacted your thoughts and feelings about your racial and cultural background?	o **Yes** o **No** o **Not sure**
If yes, please describe:	

My Goals for This Workbook

1. Check the cultural stress impacts you have had the greatest difficulty knowing how to manage or cope with.	○ Emotional stress ○ Agency stress ○ Identity stress

2. How do you hope this workbook will help improve your overall ability to cope with the cultural stress impacts you checked above?

SO, WHERE DO YOU START?

You have just clarified the ways you hope this workbook will help you learn to cope with culturally stressful events. If you feel more than one part of this book aligns with your goals, you may have the question "Where should I start?" To help with this, take a look at the guide below.

Start with Part Two: Years of talking to people like you about their experiences have revealed that the uncomfortable and intense emotions resulting from cultural stress are universal. Therefore, this is a good place to start—figure out how you've been impacted emotionally and then learn ways to take care of yourself emotionally as you continue on your journey toward empowered coping.

Choose Your Own Adventure after Part Two: After completing Part Two, use your responses in the **My Goals for This Workbook worksheet** to select the next part of the workbook you complete.

Consider completing **Part Three** if your goals focus on identifying ways to make your surroundings less culturally stressful. This might include goals related to setting boundaries with a peer or coworker, advocating for policy changes within your school or workplace, or possibly asking others to support you in changing your environment. Part Three is also appropriate for finding ways to meaningfully remain in an environment that feels culturally stressful. This might include learning how to set and pursue important goals within these environments—especially when you feel unable to reduce the level of cultural stress in that environment.

Consider completing **Part Four** if your goals are focused primarily on the internal conversation you have with yourself about your racial and cultural background. This might include goals of wanting to better understand what it means to be from your racial and cultural background or wanting to more confidently express and share who you are with the world around you. Part Four is also appropriate for helping you experience more self-love, self-confidence, and cultural pride—even when faced with negative and hurtful messages from the people around you.

Part Five Is for Putting It All Together: In **Part Five**, you will be supported in summarizing all that you have learned from Parts Two through Four, and then learn strategies for putting all of your learning into action in whatever moment you are in. Imagine that Parts Two through Four are like skill-building drills within a sports practice—you familiarize yourself with the technique and practice each skill in isolation so that you can feel more comfortable with the skill. However, every sports team has to scrimmage for its players to put all their skills together in real time and real competition. Part Five is designed to help you do just that—gain practice sorting through all the demands of a culturally stressful situation and then decide on the set of decisions that gives you the best chance of feeling empowered in that moment.

WHEN TO SEEK PROFESSIONAL HELP WHILE COMPLETING THIS WORKBOOK

Though your trusted navigators (identified on page 6) can be an amazing resource, there are times when the impacts from cultural stress may warrant additional support from a mental health professional. Actually, you don't have to be struggling greatly or in significant need to benefit from seeing such a professional. Sometimes it is just nice to talk to someone who is knowledgeable about this topic and who is outside of your normal social circle. However, if the obstacles created by cultural stress and the emotional pain it brings are causing you to (1) struggle to achieve your goals in school or at work, (2) feel unwilling or unable to maintain your relationships, or (3) broadly feel emotionally overwhelmed for days, weeks, or maybe even months without relief, working with a mental health professional while you complete this workbook is extremely important.

Particularly, consider seeking support from a mental health professional if your cultural stress impacts include any of the following:

- Experiencing nightmares or unwanted, distressing thoughts related to experiences with cultural stress
- Feeling easily startled, often vigilant, and guarded due to experiences related to cultural stress
- Experiencing significant anxiety related to experiences with cultural stress that makes it hard for you to participate in activities or pursue goals
- Experiencing deep sadness and a difficulty experiencing enjoyment in your daily life due to experiences related to cultural stress
- Having trouble with concentrating, sleeping, or relaxing due to experiences related to cultural stress
- Broadly experiencing any thoughts, emotions, or behaviors related to experiences with cultural stress that are getting in the way of you living an enjoyable and fulfilling daily life

Additional support beyond this workbook for any of the experiences above can be obtained through the Therapy Resources at the back of the book.

Chapter 3: Recap and Reflect

RECAP

- The rest of this workbook is divided into four parts—Part Two: How to Heal and Cope with Emotional Stress; Part Three: How to Boost Your Sense of Agency and Control; Part Four: How to Cope with Identity Stress; and Part Five: Putting the Pieces of Empowered Coping Together!
- It is recommended you continue your journey through this workbook by starting with Part Two: How to Heal and Cope with Emotional Stress.
- Next, use your responses to the Cultural Stress Impact Questionnaire on pages 45–46 to help you choose between Part Three: How to Boost Your Sense of Agency and Control and Part Four: How to Cope with Identity Stress.
- Conclude with Part Five: Putting the Pieces of Empowered Coping Together! to help you strengthen your empowered coping abilities.

REFLECT

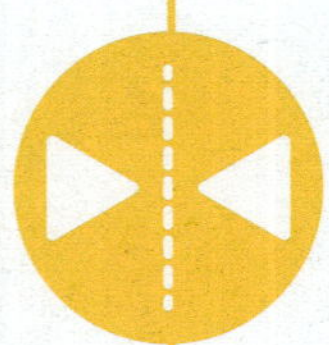

Earlier in this chapter, you were asked to identify any goals you hope to achieve while completing this workbook. Use the reflection prompts below to make sure the goals you have for this workbook are specific enough for you to notice your progress.

Are there any specific relationships or community spaces where you want to feel more confident in your ability to cope with cultural stress? If so, describe below:

What do you think you would notice yourself doing differently if you felt more confident in your coping? In other words, how would you know that you feel more confident in your ability to cope with cultural stress?

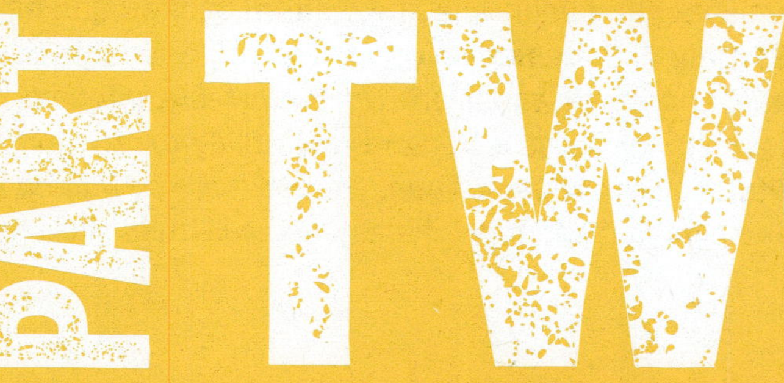

PART TWO

How to Heal and Cope with Emotional Stress

Culturally stressful events can trigger anxiety, rage, sadness, despair, and hopelessness. Sometimes these emotional reactions feel like a tidal wave rushing over you—all-consuming and inescapable. Other times, these uncomfortable emotions may be more subtle. It may be difficult to pinpoint exactly what you're feeling. Possibly the only reason you know you've been impacted is that you notice a vague sense of "I feel off today" or "That just gave me bad vibes." In either case, the impact can linger for days, weeks, or even months. You may even struggle to figure out how to heal from these emotional injuries.

In Part Two, you have the opportunity to explore the emotional stress experienced when you suspect that your race and cultural background has caused you to be mistreated, judged, or denied an opportunity. Emotional stress involves having both *uncomfortable body sensations* and *uncomfortable emotions.* The first step in learning to cope with emotional stress is to hone your ability to recognize you are experiencing this type of cultural stress impact. Then, you will learn how to be kind to yourself during this often overwhelming discomfort. Finally, you will build skills to help you heal and cope.

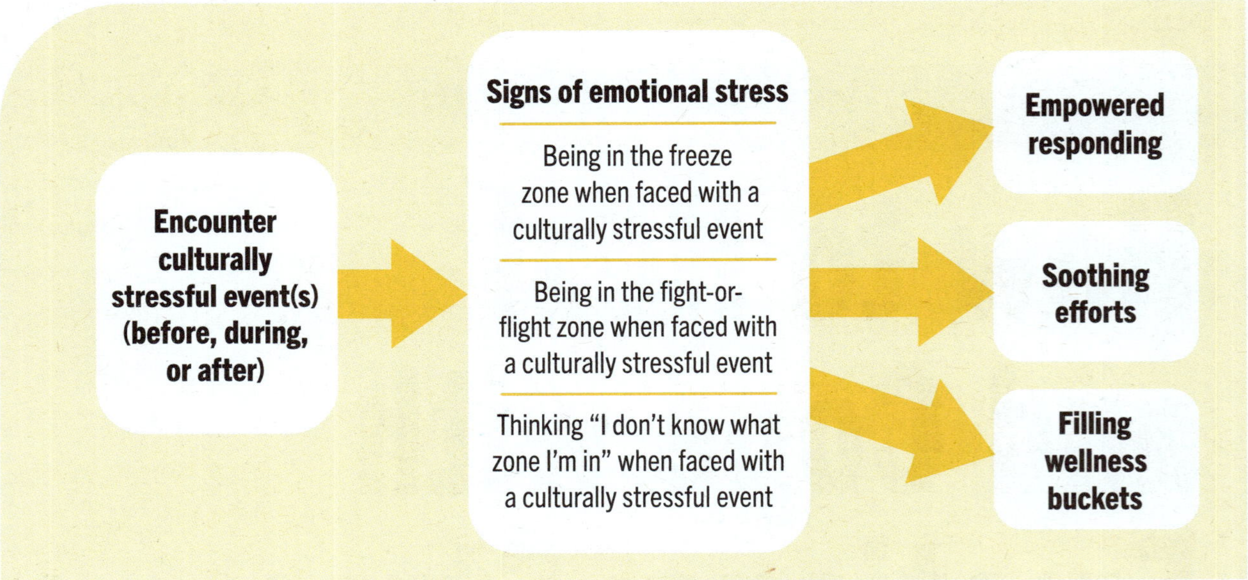

4 Noticing Emotional Stress

It's not always easy to know what emotional stress may look and feel like for you. That's because it's natural to go through the day without pausing to express curiosity toward your internal reactions to situations. You might feel a twinge of discomfort and brush it off. Choosing to take in these moments is important, because doing so can help you better understand any emotional impact a situation is having on you. That twinge may have been a sign of feeling hopelessness, sadness, or anger. Paying attention to these feelings can help you choose how you want to respond to the situation. Making empowered, wise decisions based on an accurate assessment of the emotional impact of an experience is discussed in detail later in Part Two.

It all starts with noticing the emotional stress you're experiencing. How do you do that? By practicing **mindfulness,** which involves choosing to observe and describe your body sensations, emotions, action urges, and thoughts at any given moment. In this book, these aspects of your experience are summed up as your **BEAT** (your body sensations, emotions, actions/urges, and thoughts).

TAKE YOUR BEAT

On the next page is the **BEAT diagram** you'll use throughout this workbook to help you strengthen your mindfulness skills and fully understand the emotional impact of culturally stressful events (a version for you to fill out appears later in the chapter). Taking your BEAT is a bit like taking your temperature when you feel a cold or flu coming on. It helps you figure out how your body feels, what emotions are arising, what you're thinking, and what action you feel an urge to take. That information then tells you what to do about it. When you practice taking your BEAT after culturally stressful events, it can keep the impact of cultural stress from building up without your noticing. Taking your BEAT before, during, or after a culturally stressful event can also help you fully notice its impact on you and figure out how to navigate that situation (or other similar situations) effectively.

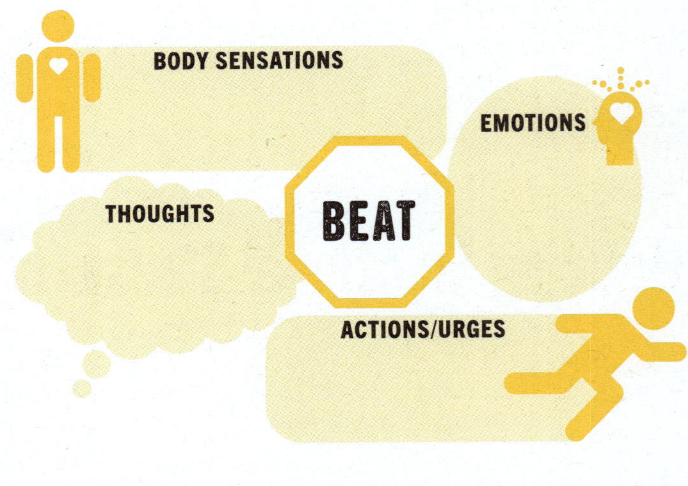

Here are the questions to ask when filling out a BEAT diagram:

1. **What body sensations are you feeling?** Muscle tension? Headache? A pit in your stomach? A heavy heart? Write down anything that you notice (including pleasant feelings, like a sense of lightness in your chest).

2. **What emotions are coming up?** Fear? Anger? Disappointment? Sorrow? All kinds of emotions may come up in response to a culturally stressful event, sometimes several at once. Give yourself a little time to try to name each emotion you are feeling—one at a time. If you find it difficult to label your emotions, you may find it helpful to search online for "Emotion Wheels" and use those diagrams to give you a menu of emotion words to choose from as you practice paying attention to your emotions.

3. **What action urges do you feel?** Do you want to exit the building, turn away, strike out, yell, mumble something, freeze, laugh? It is important that you learn to catch an action urge ("I want to quit my job") before engaging in the action ("I quit my job"). Noticing your urges will help you choose whether acting on an urge will or will not be helpful for you.

4. **What are you thinking?** That you're being treated unfairly? That you're never going to be able to reach your goals facing these obstacles? Thoughts can easily be confused with emotions. A thought is "I feel like today is going to be a good day." While emotions can be described using one-word labels ("I feel happy" or "I feel scared"), thoughts tend be more of an inner dialogue or self-talk about ourselves or the world around us. Also, our thoughts can be about the past ("Yesterday was a good day"), the present ("Today is a good day"), or the future ("Tomorrow will be a good day").

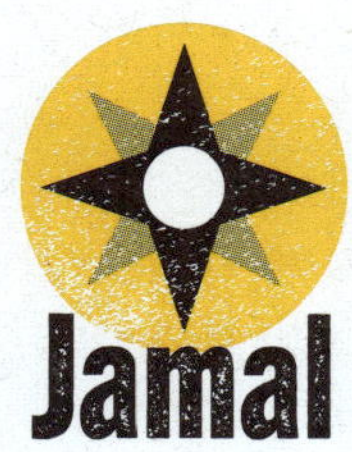

Jamal's BEAT after an Exhausting Start to the Workweek

In Chapter 3, you got a snapshot of a Monday in Jamal's work life. Now he's back home, exhausted following a series of culturally stressful experiences: uncertainty of why the women crossed the street instead of walking alongside him, having attended a meeting where his White coworkers debated whether police brutality was a real threat to the Black community, learning he may be at a disadvantage for the promotion he's been working hard to get, and being expected to assume responsibility for leading his company's antiracism initiative. Jamal used the BEAT diagram to practice mindfulness after he got home. As he sat on his couch, he noticed how physically exhausted he felt. He became aware of how his body felt tired and noticed his eyes struggling to stay open. He described feeling a bit sad and hopeless, noting thoughts like "I don't know how much more of this I can take." Jamal described the urge to start looking for a new job.

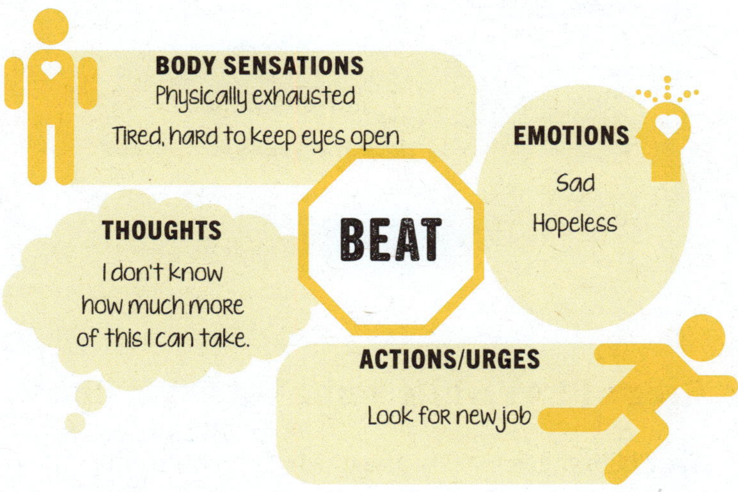

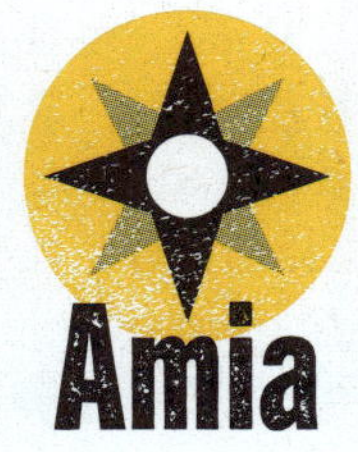

Amia's BEAT before Interacting with a Classmate Who Made Her Uncomfortable

Amia just learned that she has been paired with Thomas, a White male student, for a class project. Amia has overheard others talking about how Thomas and his friends don't believe the students of color in their class are smart and Thomas doesn't like working with them. While walking up to Thomas's desk, she sees Thomas look her way, make a comment to his friend, and then Thomas and his friend start laughing. But just when Amia reaches Thomas, he and his friend stop laughing and Thomas asks Amia, "Are you ready to get to work?"

Amia used the BEAT diagram to practice mindfulness before interacting with Thomas. She noticed that her neck and shoulders became tense, she became sweaty, and her stomach felt like it was in knots. As she walked toward him, she felt anxious and fearful, as she noticed thoughts of "I don't want to say the wrong thing or make a mistake, or else I'll prove them right." Her body sensations, emotions, and thoughts led Amia to have the urge to tell the teacher she felt unwell so that she could go to the nurse's office and possibly even be sent home.

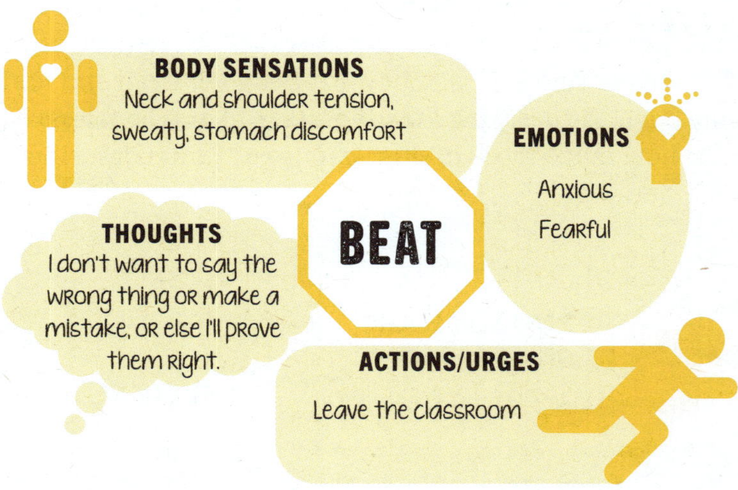

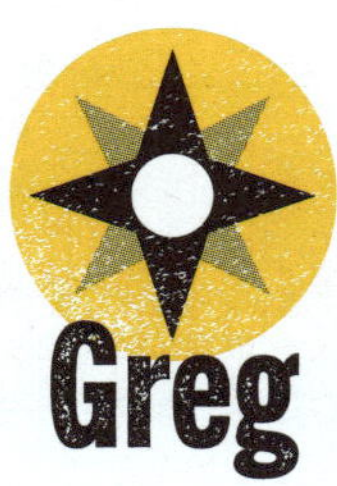

Greg's BEAT while Being Teased in Class

Greg is in math class—one of his favorite subjects—studying algebra. His teacher asks if anyone knows how to solve the equation on the board. Greg enthusiastically raises his hand and answers the question correctly. After receiving praise from the teacher, his Black and Latino peers next to him begin to tease him: "You are such a teacher's pet." He also overhears them mocking his voice and then stating, "He wants so bad to be like the White kids across town." Greg used the BEAT diagram to practice mindfulness in the moment right after hearing his classmates teasing him about his class participation. He noticed tension in his hands and his body getting warmer. While sitting at his desk, he felt angry and noticed thoughts of "I am tired of getting picked on for doing my thing in the classroom." All of this caused Greg to feel the urge to yell at his classmates and say, "Y'all are just mad cuz y'all are too dumb to even know what's going on."

BODY SENSATIONS
Hands clenching
Warmer body
EMOTIONS
Anger
THOUGHTS
I am tired of getting picked on for doing my thing in the classroom.
BEAT
ACTIONS/URGES
Yelling

YOUR TURN

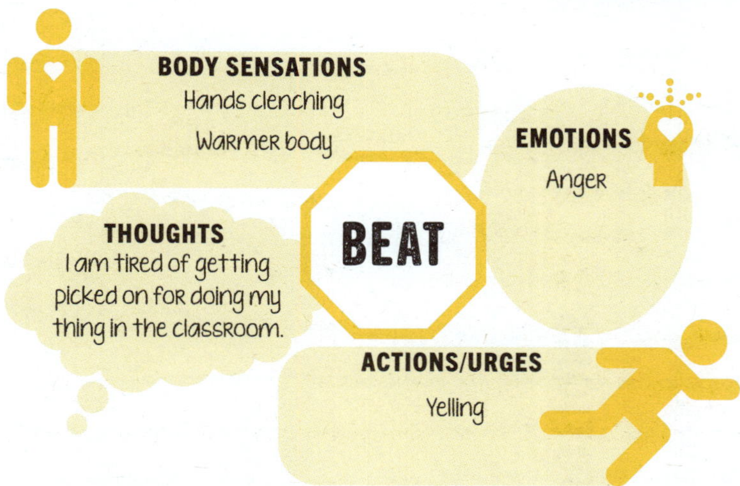

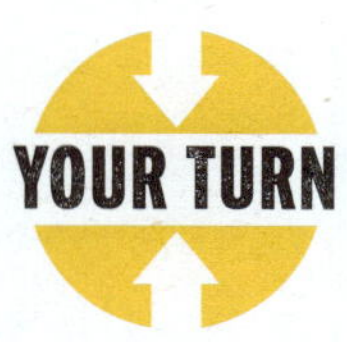

Now that you've seen how our navigators used mindfulness to notice the emotional impact of a culturally stressful event—before, during, and after—try mindfulness right now for yourself. Observe and describe your body sensations, emotions, action urges, and thoughts *in this moment*. Your BEAT diagram (see page 58) may include reactions to the navigators' stories or reactions to something else going on around you in this moment.

Power Up! Tips for Boosting Your Empowered Coping

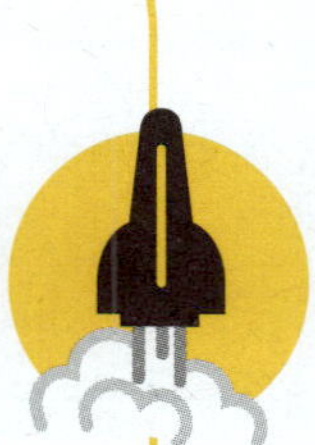

If you notice that it's hard to fill in your BEAT diagram right now, that's okay. You will get more practice doing so in the rest of the chapter. Also, here are some additional exercises to help boost your ability to take a BEAT:

- **Be a mindful participant.** Find an enjoyable and low-stress activity, like eating a favorite food, listening to your favorite song, or hanging with your closest friends. Then, during this activity, try to pause every few moments and check in with your BEAT by asking questions like "What emotions do I feel in this moment?" or "What kinds of action urges are coming up for me in this moment?
- **Journal.** Take a few moments to freely write down your reactions to a recent event. Then, after about 5–10 minutes, pause and use the BEAT diagram to help you look for examples of body sensations, emotions, action urges, or thoughts in your journaling.
- **Express yourself artistically.** For some, artistic expressions, like writing poetry, songwriting, or drawing, are ways they express their BEATs. If creative and artistic expressions are some of the strengths you listed in your Who Am I? diagram (see page 14), consider using the BEAT diagram to help notice if your art captures any of the body sensations, emotions, action urges, or thoughts you are having in a given a moment.

My BEAT

BODY SENSATIONS

EMOTIONS

THOUGHTS

BEAT

ACTIONS/URGES

CATEGORIZE YOUR EMOTIONAL STRESS

As shown by our navigators, emotional stress can occur before, during, or after a stressful situation and can include a variety of uncomfortable body sensations, emotions, and action urges. To help you use your mindfulness skills to notice when emotional stress is impacting your daily life, I created **emotional stress zones,** summarized in the following chart. The chart shows how our thoughts about a particular relationship or part of our community can cause us to experience different types of emotional stress. Take a few moments to read about each zone in the chart before reading on.

<table>
<tr><th></th><th></th><th>BODY SENSATION</th><th>EMOTION</th><th>ACTION URGE</th></tr>
<tr><td rowspan="2">EMOTIONAL STRESS ZONES</td><td>FREEZE ZONE
(Ongoing Threat/ Aftermath)</td><td>Body numbness
Dissociation*
Decreased
○ Heart rate
○ Breathing
*Dissociation is feeling disconnected from your body, thoughts, or sense of self</td><td>○ Depression
○ Numb
○ Hopeless
○ Helpless
○ Shame
○ Guilt</td><td rowspan="2">○ Avoiding people/places
○ Aggressive/confrontative
○ Vigilant/watchful
○ Social withdrawal
○ Isolation
○ Giving up on goals
○ Distraction seeking
○ Hiding identity
○ Doom scrolling*
○ Sleeping more/less
○ Eating more/less
○ Substance use
○ Work harder
○ Activism
○ Hiding emotions
*Doom scrolling is the urge to research gruesome details about violent or shocking events</td></tr>
<tr><td>FIGHT-OR-FLIGHT ZONE
(Detected Threat)</td><td>Increased
○ Heart rate
○ Breathing
○ Muscle tension
○ Stomach discomfort
○ Shakiness</td><td>○ Frustration
○ Worry/Nervous
○ Anger
○ Panic/Fear</td></tr>
<tr><td></td><td>SAFE AND SECURE ZONE</td><td>Typical
○ Heart rate
○ Breathing
Rested
Better concentration</td><td>○ Curious
○ Calm
○ Joy
○ Content
○ Love (self/others)</td><td>○ Socially engaged
○ Exploring
○ Mindful Participation</td></tr>
</table>

SAFE AND SECURE ZONE

At the bottom of the chart is the **safe and secure zone.** While it's impossible to feel relaxed 24 hours/7 days a week, the hope is that we can find safety and security within at least some relationships and some parts of our community. Often we find ourselves in this zone when we feel free from cultural stress, protected from emotional or physical harm, or surrounded by people and places that help us confidently express who we are. One way to know that you feel safe and secure is by pausing, observing, and noticing that your body feels calm and you're able to experience comfortable (or at times even positive) emotions within a relationship or while spending time in a part of your community. In such moments, you may find yourself able to focus better and meaningfully engage in activities, like having a conversation, completing a project, or simply hanging out with friends.

FIGHT-OR-FLIGHT ZONE

One step up in the chart is the **fight-or-flight zone.** Have you ever heard of the body's *fight-or-flight reaction?* When you sense an oncoming threat, like feeling as if you may be mistreated or judged unfairly due to your identity, your body readies you to face such a challenge. Interestingly, you may have this reaction whether the threat is physical (someone trying to harm your body) or social (someone judging you negatively because of your identity). Often, a detected threat is a detected threat. Also, over time and after repeated experiences of cultural stress, *the fight-or-flight reaction can activate even with the slightest reminder of past cultural stress*—like Amia becoming immediately anxious if she were paired with Thomas again in the future. One way to know that you're in the fight-or-flight zone is by noticing your body sensations becoming more activated—possibly your heart beats faster, your body temperature changes, or your breathing becomes shallower. Along with these body sensations, this zone includes feeling worried or nervous that you may experience cultural stress, like what Amia felt before working with Thomas. Or it could include feeling angry that you are presently experiencing cultural stress, like Greg while he was being judged for his class participation. In either case, this zone is nicknamed after the action urges we get in response to the detected threat—our urges often reflect a desire to *escape* or *attack* as a way of protecting ourselves from impacts of cultural stress. *Escape* urges can include avoiding or leaving uncomfortable situations or using food, video gaming, books, or substances to escape the emotional discomfort we feel from cultural stress. *Attack* urges can include becoming confrontational or yelling at the person causing cultural stress or possibly choosing to fight back with your work ethic or efforts to correct the injustices surrounding you.

FREEZE ZONE

At the top of the chart is the **freeze zone.** This zone describes instances where the intensity of your body sensations and emotions feels immobilizing, making it hard to think, feel, or choose any course of action. This most often occurs when you:

- *Feel stress that doesn't go away,* meaning you repeatedly experience cultural stress despite making many efforts to cope with the stress
- *Feel sudden or unexpected stress,* meaning you're caught off guard with seemingly no time to prepare for the intense emotional discomfort a stressful situation causes
- *Deal with the aftermath from a culturally stressful experience,* meaning you can feel, like Jamal, run down, unsure of what to do, or unsure what you have left to give

One way to know you're in the freeze zone is by pausing and observing your body sensations in moments when you feel caught up in repeated experiences of cultural stress, unexpectedly impacted by cultural stress, or immediately after experiencing cultural stress. You may notice then that it's hard to detect what's going on in your body. You may feel shocked or even unsure what to feel in these moments. Or your body may feel numb or as if you can't feel sensations as fully as usual.

Importantly, feeling numb or disconnected from the body is a common response to experiencing repeated physical or social threats over the course of time—it's another way your body tries to protect you from overwhelming moments of stress. And, when in the freeze zone, you may notice emotional states that seem to linger for extended periods of time, such as deep sadness (or depression), hopelessness, guilt, or shame. As this zone's nickname suggests, you can experience action urges that reflect feeling stuck or a lack of agency, such as wanting to give up on tasks, hide your identity, separate yourself from people, or avoid activities that you typically enjoy.

HOW TO KNOW WHEN YOU'RE EXPERIENCING EMOTIONAL STRESS

Many events and situations, including mistreatment due to your identity, can have a strong emotional impact. But when does "impact" become "stress"? This is where your BEAT diagram is key. Here are the steps for using your BEAT reaction to know when you're under significant emotional stress:

1. **Describe the culturally stressful situation.** Where were you? Who was there? What relationship or community stressor arose?
2. **Use the BEAT diagram to label your physical sensations, emotions, thoughts, and actions/urges.**
3. **Describe the impact of the culturally stressful event.** Do you notice any of the

three indicators of emotional stress (described below) when looking at your BEAT reaction?

- **"I am in the freeze zone."** It's natural to experience some uncomfortable body sensations or emotional responses to culturally stressful events. But several BEAT reactions that feature feelings of shame, guilt, hopelessness, or sadness over several days or maybe even weeks can be a sign that you may benefit from exploring options to cope with emotional stress. This is especially important if you also notice yourself struggling to maintain efforts toward meaningful life goals, like attending school, completing schoolwork, continuing to spend time with friends, or even maintaining daily hygiene routines.

- **"I am in the fight-or-flight zone."** Are you feeling more vigilant and watchful for possible culturally stressful events? Becoming extremely anxious or even angry when anticipating or first confronted with such experiences? In either case, you may notice, looking back, that you're using coping methods that really aren't helping you emotionally. Maybe you even notice your coping responses are actually disruptive and causing problems in other areas of your life, like you're getting in trouble for your confrontation, your grades are suffering because of your avoidance, or you're becoming concerningly dependent on substances. These are all signs that focusing on building your emotional stress coping skills may be beneficial.

- **"I don't know what zone I'm in."** Culturally stressful events can have a confusing impact. If you're not used to paying attention to your emotions, it can be hard to know exactly what you're feeling. Or, even with decent mindfulness skills and familiarity with what culturally stressful events typically look and feel like, you're sometimes left speechless, confused, and uncertain about the emotional impact of a specific event. Think of these moments as opportunities to use the BEAT diagram and emotional stress zones chart to help you check in with yourself. Doing so may help you notice emotional stress early and help you thoughtfully select coping responses that support your healing.

IDENTIFY EMOTIONAL STRESS

Moving forward, you can use the **Identifying My Emotional Stress worksheet** on page 64 to help you pause, notice, and label the signs of emotional stress any time you are curious about whether you are experiencing (or have experienced) emotional stress in response to a culturally stressful event(s). Greg followed the steps above to fill out his worksheet, shown on the facing page.

Greg

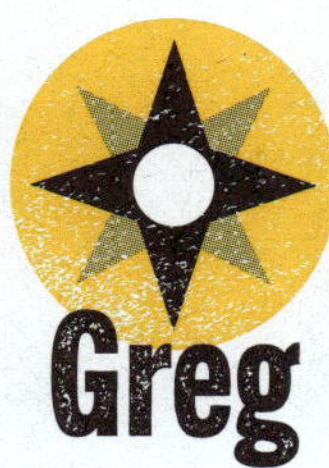

Greg's Emotional Stress

Earlier in this chapter, you read about Greg's reactions to culturally stressful interactions with his classmates. Here is how Greg used this worksheet.

1. Describe the culturally stressful situation.

☐ Where are you?	Math class
☐ Who was present?	My class and teacher. Sitting near my friends
☐ Describe the relationship or community stressor	Being judged for caring about school and participating

2. Use the BEAT diagram to label your physical sensations, emotions, thoughts, and actions/urges.

BODY SENSATIONS
Hands clenching
Warmer body
EMOTIONS
Anger
BEAT
THOUGHTS
I am tired of getting picked on for doing my thing in the classroom.
ACTIONS/URGES
Yelling

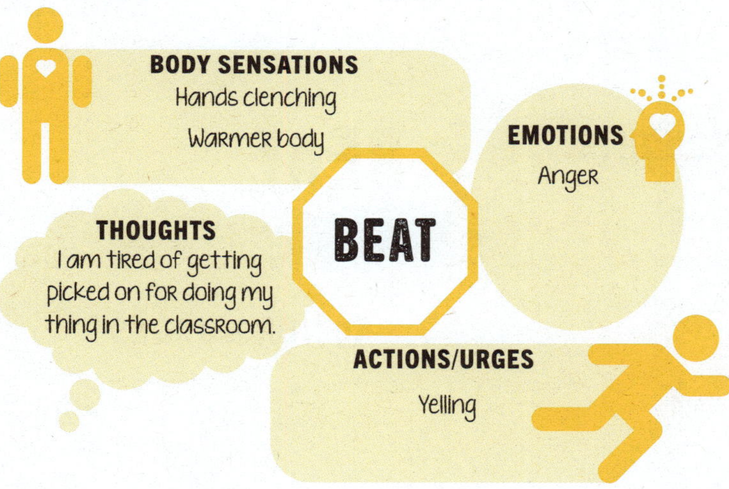

3. Describe the impact of the culturally stressful event. When looking at your BEAT diagram, do you notice yourself having any of the following impacts?

"I am in the freeze zone."	○ Yes ● No
"I am in the fight-or-flight zone."	● Yes ○ No
"I don't know what zone I'm in."	○ Yes ● No

Identifying My Emotional Stress

1. Describe the culturally stressful situation.

Where are you?	
Who was present?	
Describe the relationship or community stressor	

2. Use the BEAT diagram to label your physical sensations, emotions, thoughts, and actions/urges.

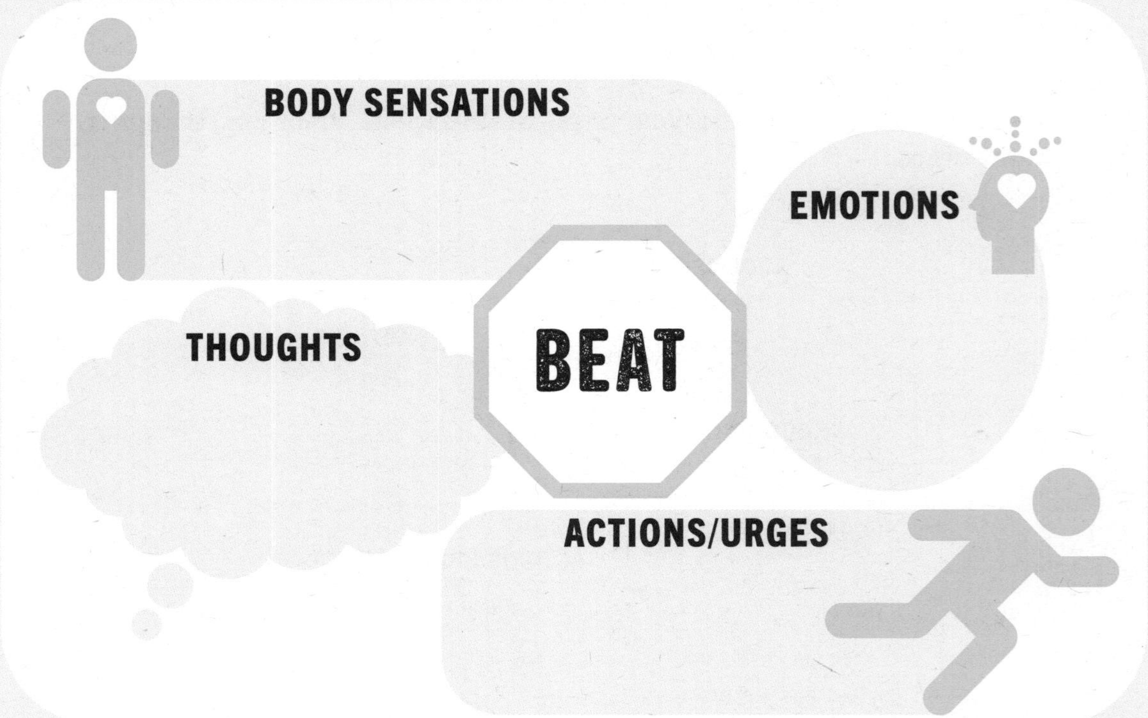

BODY SENSATIONS

EMOTIONS

THOUGHTS

BEAT

ACTIONS/URGES

3. Describe the impact of the culturally stressful event. When looking at your BEAT diagram, do you notice your reactions falling in any of the zones below?

"I am in the freeze zone."	o Yes o No
"I am in the fight-or-flight zone."	o Yes o No
"I don't know what zone I'm in."	o Yes o No

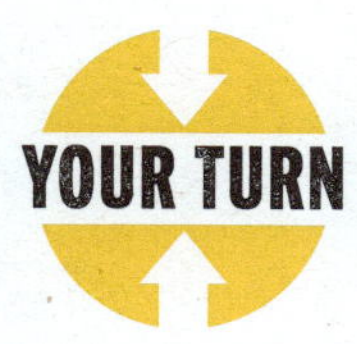

Now fill in each step of the Identifying My Emotional Stress worksheet (on the facing page), as Greg did.

Power Up! Tips for Boosting Your Empowered Coping

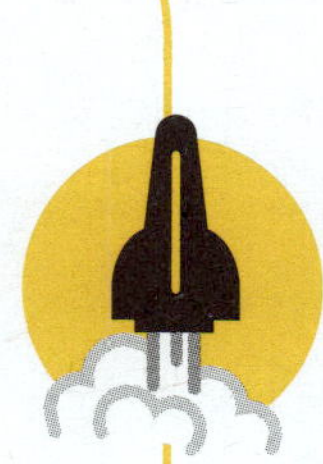

- If you indicated "yes" for any of these indicators, consider using the emotional stress coping diagram in Chapter 6 (see page 80).
- If you're having trouble sticking with uncomfortable feelings long enough to identify them, try to combine taking a BEAT with some of the coping skills introduced in Chapter 8. Possibly, spend a few seconds or minutes observing and describing your BEAT reactions followed by engaging in a soothing activity, such as a breathing exercise.

Chapter 4: Recap and Reflect

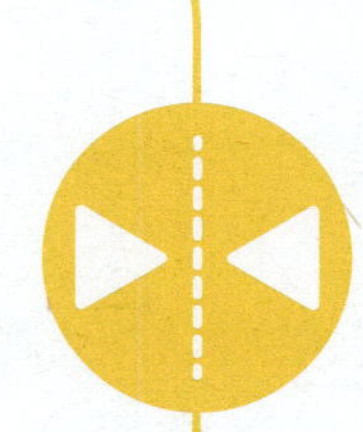

RECAP

- **Mindfulness** involves choosing to pause, observe, and describe body sensations, emotions, action urges, and thoughts at any given moment.
- You can use the **BEAT diagram** to help you observe and describe these parts of your experience.
- To help you identify emotional stress when you're experiencing it, you can use the BEAT diagram to observe if you're in either of the **emotional stress zones** (*fight-or-flight zone* or *freeze zone).*

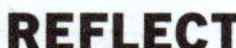

REFLECT

Now that you're more familiar with what emotional stress looks and feels like, record in the **My Experiences in Emotional Stress Zones worksheet** (on the next page) a time when you were in the freeze, fight-or-flight, or safe and secure zone and then describe your BEAT reactions to this situation.

My Experiences in Emotional Stress Zones

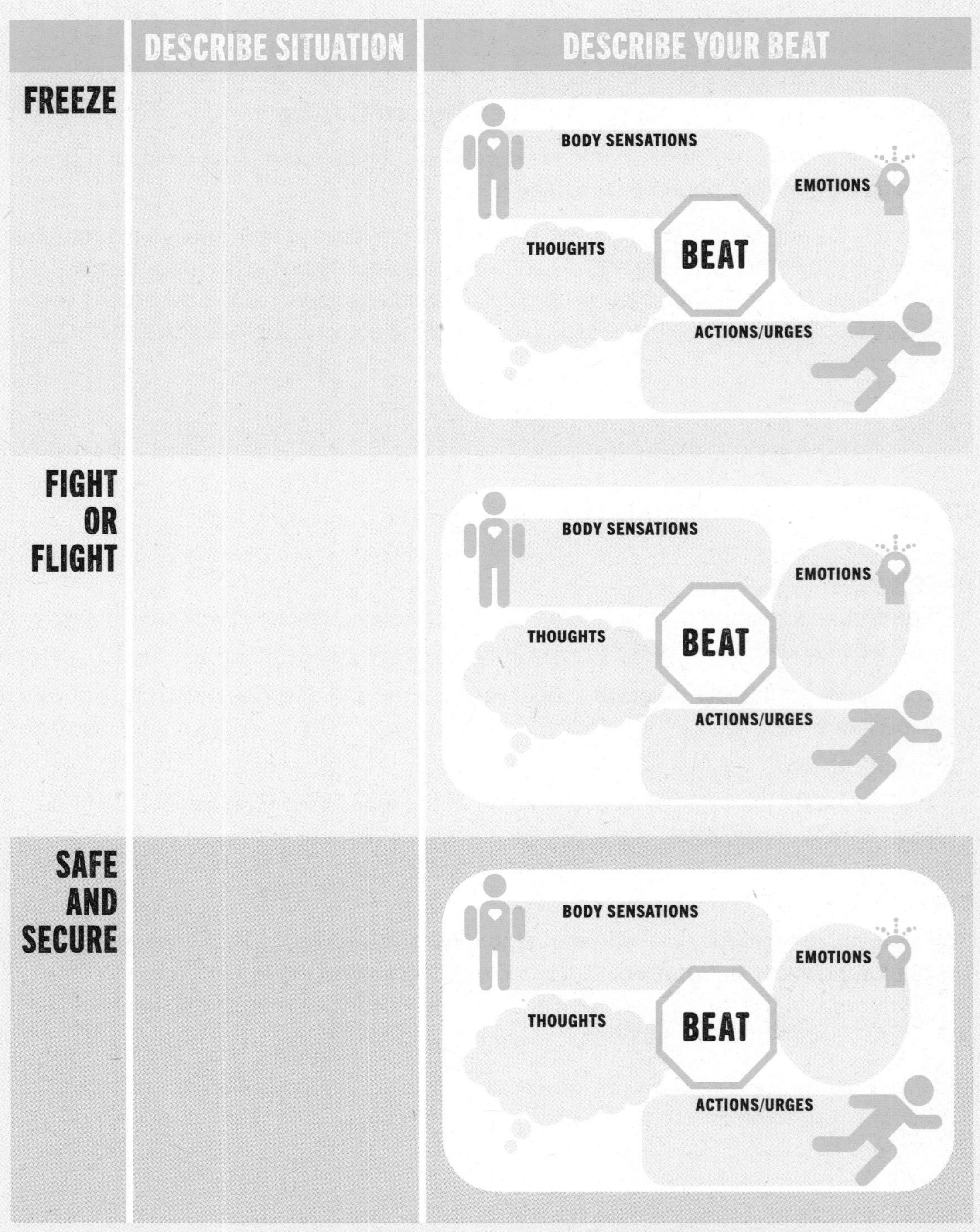

5 How Can I Show Kindness and Understanding toward My Emotional Stress?

When using the BEAT diagram to notice any emotional stress, it's also important to pay attention to your thoughts and feelings about the BEAT reaction you're having. I know that sounds a little weird—noticing your reaction to your reaction sounds kind of meta, right? Think about it this way. On TV shows, there is a main character who often experiences all types of emotions as they run into different situations during an episode. And then, on some shows, there is a narrator—you know, the background voice that reacts to and comments on the main character's responses to the situations they face. Such a narrator could be understanding and empathetic toward the main character's feelings about their circumstance. For example, imagine a narrator who uses a gentle and tender voice while saying—"She feels a slight sadness and a tear gently runs down her cheek as her parents drive away." This type of narration warmly acknowledges and describes the main character's emotional experience.

Away from our screens, many of us have a different and at times louder narrator. One that is quite critical and judgmental toward our emotional expression. Imagine this narrator's voice to be stern and yelling, "What's wrong with you? Toughen up and stop being so sensitive." Such narration can make it difficult to cope with our emotions and can even encourage us to go to great lengths to avoid the emotions we feel. In real life, we are both the main character living our stories and the narrator commenting on them.

As your own main character, you can use mindfulness to observe and describe your BEAT reactions at any point of your story. **Self-compassion,** however, describes choosing to turn up the volume on the understanding and loving narrator while trying to turn your focus away from the critical and judgmental narrator.

In this chapter you'll learn a few skills for showing kindness and understanding toward yourself during moments of emotional stress. Specifically, you will gain skills for noticing any self-judgments that are coming from the overly critical narrator. Then you'll learn strategies for turning up the volume on your compassionate narrator.

STEPS FOR SHOWING KINDNESS AND UNDERSTANDING TOWARD YOUR EMOTIONAL STRESS

As described in Chapter 4, you can use the BEAT diagram to practice mindfulness and help you determine whether you've experienced emotional stress. A next move toward coping is to offer yourself some kindness for and understanding toward what you're experiencing. Here are the steps to practicing the skill of self-compassion:

1. **Catch your self-judgments.** The emotions you experience every day have a purpose. They are a representation of how you are making sense of the world around you, and they help you understand how certain situations are impacting you. But keeping this in mind can be very, very, very challenging when experiencing uncomfortable and intense body sensations and emotions. Rather, your natural response to these BEAT reactions can be quite critical and judgmental—at times, even suggesting that your reactions do not make sense or have no purpose. So, before you turn up the volume on your compassionate narrator, it can be helpful to notice any ways your critical narrator is trying to get in the way of the kindness and understanding you're hoping to express toward yourself. The table below gives a few examples of critical judgments you may have toward your emotional stress (a version for you to fill in appears later in the chapter).

TYPES OF SELF-JUDGMENT	DESCRIPTION	EXAMPLES
Critical labeling	Using labels to criticize or negatively judge yourself for having your emotional reactions to a culturally stressful event (*Hint:* You may be experiencing this self-judgment if you use "I am" thinking.)	Because of the emotions I experience: • "*I am* so weak." • "*I am* soft." • "*I am* emotionally sensitive." • "*I am* too reactive."
Self-blame	Feeling as if your uncomfortable emotions suggest that you have done something wrong or that you need to do something better (*Hint:* You may be experiencing this self-judgment if your thoughts are focusing more on yourself and what you did or did not do.)	"If I had spoken up for myself, I wouldn't be feeling so bad right now." "It has nothing to do with them. I'm feeling this way because I didn't work hard enough." "I need to learn to suck it up and just deal with it."

TYPES OF SELF-JUDGMENT	DESCRIPTION	EXAMPLES
Oversimplified coping	Assuming you should be able to quickly get over, forget about, or stop the emotional stress you are feeling (*Hint:* You may be experiencing this self-judgment if you are using "should" thinking.)	"It's not like I'm surprised this happened. I *shouldn't* feel this upset." "I *should* have tougher skin." "I know they just want to get me upset. I *shouldn't* have reacted that way."

2. Reflect on how your emotions make sense. Often we're more willing to embrace and accept what we can understand and what we feel is useful. For example, consider someone who just completed a strenuous workout and now feels sore. Though the body's soreness may be unwanted, a compassionate narrator who states, "It makes sense that my legs are sore—I just completed 50 squats and lunges," would encourage someone to be more accepting of their soreness. Also, a compassionate narrator might help differentiate soreness from other body sensations, like a sharp and concerning pain—"this soreness tells me I pushed myself today." Such an acknowledgment helps to label soreness as a sign of wellness and improving strength rather than a reason to be concerned or contact a doctor.

Just as your body sensations can communicate understandable and useful information, your emotions can be informative. Learning the language of your emotions can help you show kindness and understanding toward them. The chart below highlights the information that your emotions can provide to help you understand how your surroundings are impacting you (a version for you to fill out appears later in the chapter).

MY CURRENT EMOTIONS	WHAT TO THINK ABOUT
"I feel anxious."	Is my anxiety alerting me to feeling **unsafe, threatened, or concerned about a possible outcome?**
"I feel sad."	Is my sadness alerting me to feeling a **lack of connection, belonging, purpose, or hope, or that I am struggling to cope with a loss?**
"I feel angry."	Is my anger alerting me to feeling **disrespected, unheard, not seen, unsupported, victimized, or violated?**
"I feel guilt."	Is my guilt alerting me to **something that I did wrong or that negatively impacted someone else?**
"I feel shame."	Is my shame or embarrassment alerting me to feeling **as if I have done something that will cause me to be judged negatively or deny me the ability to be loved by or connected with others?**
"I feel loved."	Is my love alerting me to feeling **connected, taken care of, appreciated, affirmed, or supported?**

MY CURRENT EMOTIONS	WHAT TO THINK ABOUT
"I feel content."	Is my contentment alerting me to feeling **most of my important needs and/or wants are met?**
"I feel proud."	Is my pride alerting me to feeling **thankful for how my decisions, my accomplishments, or my social interactions aligned with the things I care about most in life?**
"I feel joy."	Is my joy alerting me to feeling a sense of **lightness, hope for my future, acceptance of myself, and love for myself?**
Other emotion: "I feel ________."	Is this emotion alerting me to anything important about how I am impacted by my surroundings?

3. Compassionately respond as if your emotions make sense. After reflecting on what your emotions may be communicating, take a few moments to treat your emotions as if they make sense with a compassionate response. In this chapter you will use the reflection prompts below to help you generate a compassionate response to your uncomfortable emotions (a version for you to fill in appears later in the chapter).

State your emotions	In this moment, I notice that I feel (describe your BEAT reaction below):
Acknowledge any self-judgments	In this moment, I recognize that I am feeling critical of the emotions I am experiencing in these ways:
Compassionately respond to your emotions	Though I am tempted to be critical of my emotions right now, I can try to be kind and understanding toward my emotions by saying/doing:

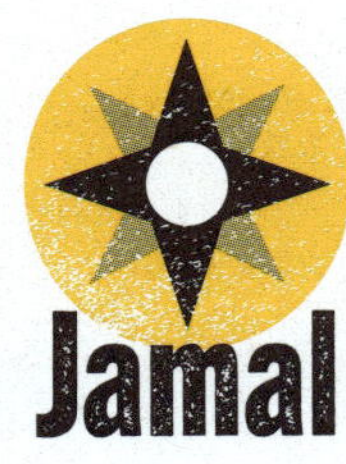

Jamal's Efforts to Show Kindness and Understanding toward His Emotional Stress

In Chapter 4, you learned about Jamal's BEAT reaction to a day involving several culturally stressful events. By completing his BEAT diagram, Jamal noticed he was experiencing body sensations and emotions that fell into the freeze zone of the emotional stress zones chart. He observed himself feeling physically run down, emotionally sad and hopeless, and as if his only option was to leave his job. Let's see how Jamal used the steps in this chapter to show kindness and understanding toward his emotional stress.

1. Catch your self-judgments. As you can see in his critical self-judgments chart on the facing page, Jamal used this step to acknowledge different ways his critical narrator was making it difficult for him to have self-compassion toward the emotional stress he was experiencing.

TYPES OF SELF-JUDGMENT	MY SELF-JUDGMENTS
Critical labeling	Because of how exhausted I feel, I guess I am someone who's not cut out for this job.
Self-blame	I feel this way because I have not done a good job with setting boundaries. I'd be feeling much better if I just stood up for myself more.
Oversimplified coping	I'm just getting started in my career. I shouldn't feel this tired and worn down.

2. Reflect on how your emotions make sense. Jamal mainly experienced sadness and hopelessness following a long workday. He was able to use this step to reflect on how these emotions, particularly his sadness, were alerting him to the fact that he doesn't feel very connected with his coworkers and has lost hope that he can attain the promotion he really wants.

MY EMOTIONS	WHAT TO THINK ABOUT	MY RESPONSE
"I feel sad."	Is my sadness alerting me to feeling a **lack of connection, belonging, purpose, or hope, or that I am struggling to cope with a loss?**	● Yes ○ No ○ Maybe

3. Compassionately respond as if your emotions make sense. By the time Jamal got to step 3, his sadness and hopelessness were still there. But he noticed that he was beginning to change his own response to these emotions. Yes, they were still uncomfortable and somewhat intense. However, he was able to use this step to turn his attention away from his self-judgments and more consistently reflect on why his emotional reactions made sense given the work culture he was in.

State your emotions	In this moment, I notice that I feel (describe your BEAT reaction below): Sad and hopeless
Acknowledge any self-judgments	In this moment, I recognize that I am feeling critical of the emotions I am experiencing in these ways: I feel like my sadness and hopelessness suggest I am not cut out for my job, or even my career.
Compassionately respond to your emotions	Though I am tempted to be critical of my emotions right now, I can try to be kind and understanding toward my emotions by saying/doing: I could remind myself that it makes sense I am feeling sad and hopeless after a day like this because I don't feel connected with anyone at my job and don't feel supported by anyone right now at my job.

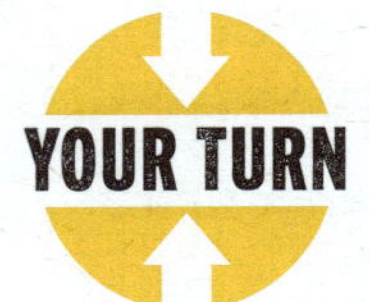

Use the prompts below to help you turn up your compassionate narrator any time you face emotional stress.

1. **Catch your self-judgments.** Describe any critical self-judgments you have toward the body sensations and emotions you are experiencing in the form on page 73.

2. **Reflect on how your emotions make sense.** Use the **What Are My Emotions Telling Me? chart** on page 74 to help you answer the question "What kind of information am I getting from my emotions in this moment?"

3. **Compassionately respond as if your emotions make sense.** Use the prompts in the **My Compassionate Response to My Emotions worksheet** on page 75 to help you compassionately show kindness and understanding toward your emotions.

Power Up! Tips for Boosting Your Empowered Coping

- **Self-compassion is not pushing away the emotion.** Try not to focus on the hope that practicing self-compassion in this way will make your emotions go away. That's not likely, and it's not the goal here. The goal is to help you find a way to show kindness and understanding toward what you're feeling while you explore additional coping decisions for the moment you are in.
- **Self-compassion is like starting a new relationship.** Expressing kindness and understanding toward yourself may be difficult at first. Some people feel uncomfortable turning up this new compassionate narrator's volume or even find this narrator hard to believe. Try thinking of building self-compassion as developing a new relationship with a part of yourself. And, just like any new relationship, this relationship you are building with yourself can feel awkward and uncomfortable. So, if you notice any feelings of awkwardness or discomfort while practicing self-compassion, remind yourself that this BEAT reaction *makes sense* and that with time and careful practice, a new, loving, and supportive relationship with your emotions can grow.
- **How would you support a friend?** Sometimes it's easier to use our friendships to help us think of ways to respond compassionately to our emotions. For example, imagine that you have a friend who is experiencing the same hurt emotions you are. Think of the ways you would try to support them. Consider the tone of voice, body language, and words you would say to help them understand that their emotions *make sense.* Consider writing down, word for word, what you might say to or do for them. After doing this, try to use the same tone, words, and actions to express kindness and understanding toward your own emotions.

My Critical Self-Judgments about My Physical Sensations and Emotions

TYPES OF SELF-JUDGMENT	DESCRIPTION	MY SELF-JUDGMENTS
Critical labeling	Using labels to criticize or negatively judge yourself for having your emotional reactions to a culturally stressful event (*Hint:* You may be experiencing this self-judgment if you use "I am" thinking.)	
Self-blame	Feeling as if your uncomfortable emotions suggest that you have done something wrong or that you need to do something better (*Hint:* You may be experiencing this self-judgment if your thoughts are focusing more on yourself and what you did or did not do.)	
Oversimplified coping	Assuming you should be able to quickly get over, forget about, or stop the emotional stress you are feeling (*Hint:* You may be experiencing this self-judgment if you are using "should" thinking.)	
Other	List any other self-judgments you might have toward your emotions in this moment:	

What Are My Emotions Telling Me?

MY EMOTIONS	WHAT TO THINK ABOUT	MY RESPONSE
"I feel anxious."	Is my anxiety alerting me to feeling **unsafe, threatened, or concerned about a possible outcome?**	○ Yes ○ No ○ Maybe
"I feel sad."	Is my sadness alerting me to feeling a **lack of connection, belonging, purpose, or hope, or that I am struggling to cope with a loss?**	○ Yes ○ No ○ Maybe
"I feel angry."	Is my anger alerting me to feeling **disrespected, unheard, not seen, unsupported, victimized, or violated?**	○ Yes ○ No ○ Maybe
"I feel guilt."	Is my guilt alerting me to **something that I did wrong or that negatively impacted someone else?**	○ Yes ○ No ○ Maybe
"I feel shame."	Is my shame or embarrassment alerting me to feeling **as if I have done something that will cause me to be judged negatively or deny me the ability to be loved by or connected with others?**	○ Yes ○ No ○ Maybe
"I feel loved."	Is my love alerting me to feeling **connected, taken care of, appreciated, affirmed, or supported?**	○ Yes ○ No ○ Maybe
"I feel content."	Is my contentment alerting me to feeling **most of my important needs and/or wants are met?**	○ Yes ○ No ○ Maybe
"I feel proud."	Is my pride alerting me to feeling **thankful for how my decisions, my accomplishments, or my social interactions aligned with the things I care about most in life?**	○ Yes ○ No ○ Maybe
"I feel joy."	Is my joy alerting me to feeling a sense of **lightness, hope for my future, acceptance of myself, and love for myself?**	○ Yes ○ No ○ Maybe
Other emotion: "I feel ___________."	Is this emotion alerting me to anything important about how I am impacted by my surroundings?	○ Yes ○ No ○ Maybe

My Compassionate Response to My Emotions

State your emotions	In this moment, I notice that I feel (describe your BEAT reaction below):
Acknowledge any self-judgments	In this moment, I recognize that I am feeling critical of the emotions I am experiencing in these ways:
Compassionately respond to your emotions	Though I am tempted to be critical of my emotions right now, I can try to be kind and understanding toward my emotions by saying/doing:

- **Compassionate responses I can use.** Because it can be hard to initially think of compassionate responses to list, here are a few compassionate responses that some teens and young adults I have worked with have used. Try them out! Or create your own compassionate response that will help you show kindness and understanding toward any uncomfortable emotions you experience.

"Life isn't always ideal so it's okay to be down sometimes."

"I know there are other people out there who have experienced something similar to me."

Create your own:

"My emotions make sense and have meaning because ________."

"Understanding and accepting my feelings are better than bottling them up because ________."

"I have a right to feel whichever way I happen to feel. It's good for me to take time and keep it real about how I'm feeling."

Create your own:

"My emotions have helped me to see that the most kind thing I could do for myself right now is ________."

Chapter 5: Recap and Reflect

RECAP

- **Self-compassion** describes your efforts to show kindness and understanding toward the body sensations, emotions, action urges, and thoughts (BEAT) you are experiencing in any given moment.
- Developing and growing your self-compassionate narrator will help you make decisions that ultimately take care of your emotions and support your healing from culturally stressful situations.

- One way to practice self-compassion when you experience emotional stress is to follow the following steps.
  1. Notice any critical judgments of your BEAT reaction.
  2. Reflect on the ways your emotions may make sense.
  3. Compassionately state how your emotions make sense for the situation you're in.

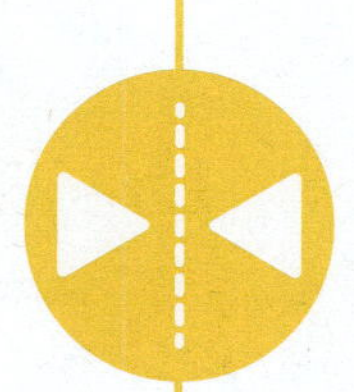

REFLECT

Before moving forward, take a moment to think about what you learned about self-compassion and how you hope this skill can help you cope with emotional stress. To do so, answer the questions below.

What does **self-compassion** mean to you, and how can it be helpful when experiencing emotional stress?

In addition to what you learned in this chapter, are there other ways that you've learned to show kindness and understanding toward your uncomfortable emotions?

How can practicing **self-compassion** enhance your ability to heal from any emotional stress you experience moving forward?

Calling in your workbook navigators: You may also find it helpful to review your answers to these questions with your workbook navigators, as you may learn some new ways to put these coping decisions into action! Specifically, your workbook navigators may be able to share instances when they have had similar emotional responses to cultural stress, help you see that your BEAT reactions are not out of the ordinary, and possibly even help you find creative ways to turn up the volume on your compassionate narrator.

6 My Emotional Stress Coping Assessment

Now that you have a better sense of how to kindly notice when you experience emotional stress, let's focus on additional ways you can cope with any uncomfortable body sensations and emotions you may feel in response to culturally stressful events. The rest of Part Two focuses on coping skills that help us "ride the wave" of emotions. Though trying to ignore or immediately eliminate our most uncomfortable emotions may seem like the best decision, doing so often causes the waves of emotion to get larger and stronger. Instead, learning to accept the reality that some emotional pain lingers, sometimes for a long time, is crucial to helping us practice empowered coping. Just as an ocean wave in motion must run its course, the kind and compassionate narrator you started to develop in Chapter 5 can remind you that you can choose to allow your emotions to do the same.

Remember, the main goal of this workbook is to help you practice empowered coping. In this case, helping you notice the emotional waves caused by cultural stress and then strengthening coping skills that help you heal from and navigate culturally stressful experiences. In this chapter, you'll have a chance to discover what you already do to ride these emotional waves and keep yourself afloat until your uncomfortable feelings subside. You'll learn to take note of any coping efforts that actually do ease the intensity of your most uncomfortable emotions in ways that do not backfire in the long run.

Also, using healthy coping skills affects the kinds of decisions you make following a culturally stressful event. If your emotions are still gnawing at you, even under the surface, your decisions can be driven by your emotional pain and may not serve you well. In this chapter, you'll also explore how you try to make sure that you will be happy with the types of decisions you make after your feelings have calmed.

HOW TO USE THE EMOTIONAL STRESS COPING DIAGRAM

The **emotional stress coping diagram** below displays three different coping skills you can use when culturally stressful events cause you to experience emotional stress. The rest of Part Two will help you practice each of these skills: making helpful decisions in the heat of the moment (Chapter 7), soothing uncomfortable body sensations and emotions as you ride the wave of emotional stress (Chapter 8), and making healthy decisions over time as you are healing from the emotional waves caused by cultural stress (Chapter 9).

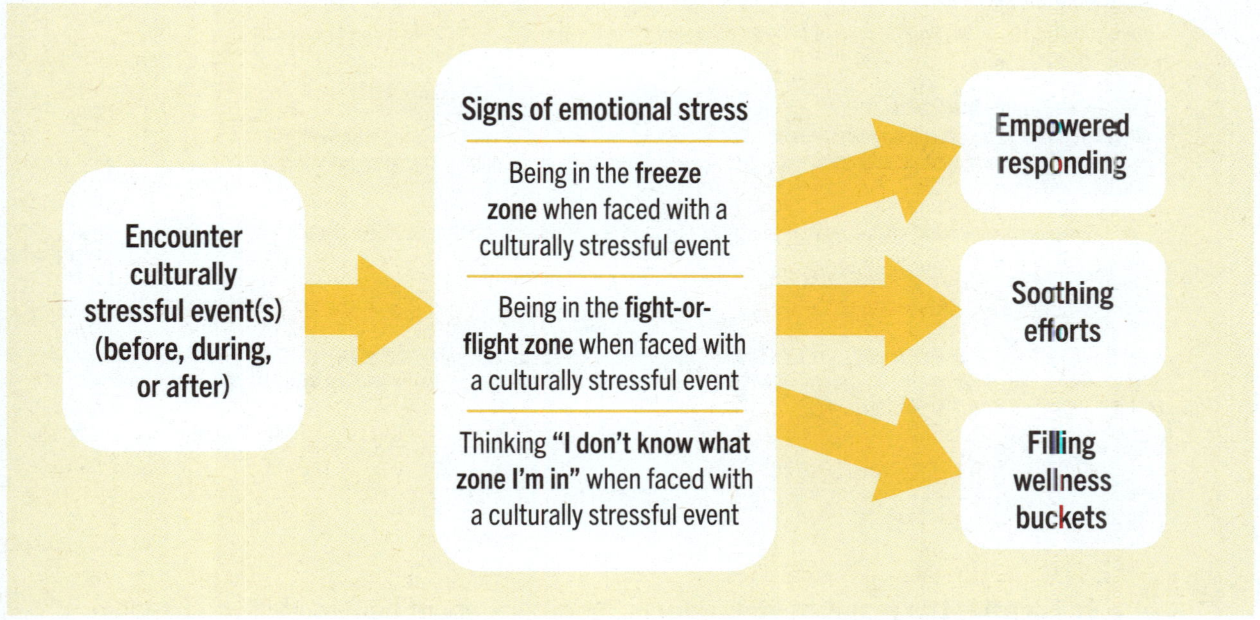

Have you already used any of these skills? Answer the questions below and see.

1. **Identify a culturally stressful event.** Describe one past, present, or anticipated culturally stressful event below that has caused you to experience emotional stress. If you have any difficulty thinking of an example, look back at your responses in Chapter 2 to help you choose one.

2. **Reflect on the emotional stress coping diagram.** Review the prompts in the next worksheet for a quick preview of each coping decision. See if you can think of examples of how you may have practiced each type of coping in response to the culturally stressful event you described above.

How Have I Been Coping with Emotional Stress?

Empowered responding Did you notice any strong action urges (like avoiding a situation, giving up, lashing out) that may have not been helpful for you to engage in?	○ Yes ○ No ○ Not sure
If "yes," were you able to resist any initial urges that you felt were unhelpful and instead engage in more helpful responses?	○ Yes ○ No ○ Not sure
Soothing efforts Were you able to use any coping skills or find any activities to soothe your uncomfortable bodily sensations and emotions?	○ Yes ○ No ○ Not sure
Filling wellness buckets While you waited for your uncomfortable body sensations and emotions to calm, were you able to keep healthy routines and continue taking care of your daily responsibilities as you healed from the culturally stressful event?	○ Yes ○ No ○ Not sure
Are there any additional ways that you try to cope with emotional stress that you have not already described?	

3. Identify the result of your efforts. Now think about how you felt you handled the emotional stress from this culturally stressful event:

Were you pleased with how you coped with your emotional stress?	○ Yes ○ No ○ Somewhat
Why or why not?	

Chapter 6: Recap and Reflect

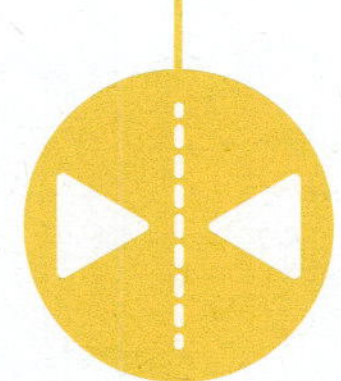

RECAP

- When you notice emotional stress, you can be tempted to look for coping strategies that quickly get rid of your discomfort.
- Instead, a more compassionate response to your emotional stress is to search for coping skills that help you ride the wave of your uncomfortable body sensations and emotions.

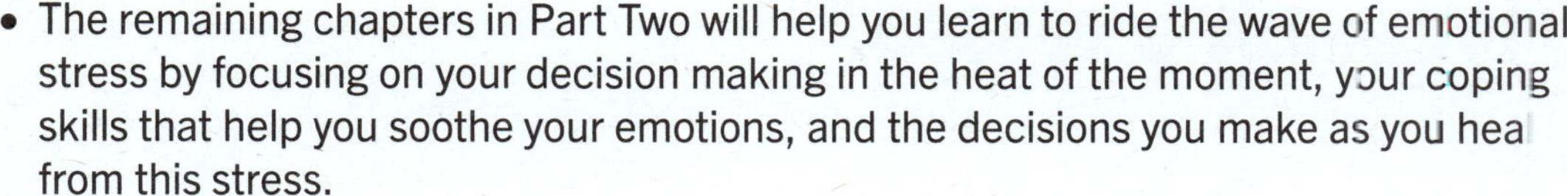

- The remaining chapters in Part Two will help you learn to ride the wave of emotional stress by focusing on your decision making in the heat of the moment, your coping skills that help you soothe your emotions, and the decisions you make as you heal from this stress.

REFLECT

Use the questionnaire below to help you determine which of the remaining chapters you are most interested in reviewing.

IMPACT FROM EMOTIONAL STRESS	RESPONSES	CHAPTER
1. Are you ever unsure how to cope with any strong and possibly unhelpful action urges you experience in the moments when emotional stress is most intense?	○ Yes ○ No	If "yes," go to Chapter 7 (on how to engage in empowered responding)
2. When faced with culturally stressful events, are you ever unsure how to soothe uncomfortable or intense body sensations or emotions?	○ Yes ○ No	If "yes," go to Chapter 8 (on how to make soothing efforts)
3. When faced with culturally stressful events, do you ever have a hard time with continuing to invest time/energy in different areas of your life?	○ Yes ○ No	If "yes," go to Chapter 9 (on how to fill wellness buckets)

7 How Can I Make Helpful Decisions in the Moment When Emotionally Stressed?

When facing the emotional waves generated by culturally stressful events, it can be hard to figure out the most helpful decisions to make in the heat of the moment. The intense, uncomfortable emotions you feel can be so distracting that all you can focus on are your immediate action urges, like urges to yell, fight back, get away, or give up. Unfortunately, if you give in to some of these immediate action urges, you later learn that such decisions have their own consequences—possibly more unwanted and uncomfortable experiences that eventually cause another rise in emotional discomfort.

Have you ever considered the difference between "reacting" versus "responding" to your most uncomfortable emotions? This chapter will help you learn to pay closer attention to the strongest action urges you experience when faced with culturally stressful events. And, instead of *reacting* without consideration for the long-term benefits or costs of your actions, you will learn to practice a skill called **empowered responding.** This coping skill encourages you to make decisions in the heat of the moment that feel meaningful and helpful to you before, during, and after facing cultural stress. You'll learn how to identify which action urges you may want to give in to and which urges might be the most important to resist. Think of this chapter as training you in this important skill now so it hopefully lightens this heavy mental lifting in the heat of the moment.

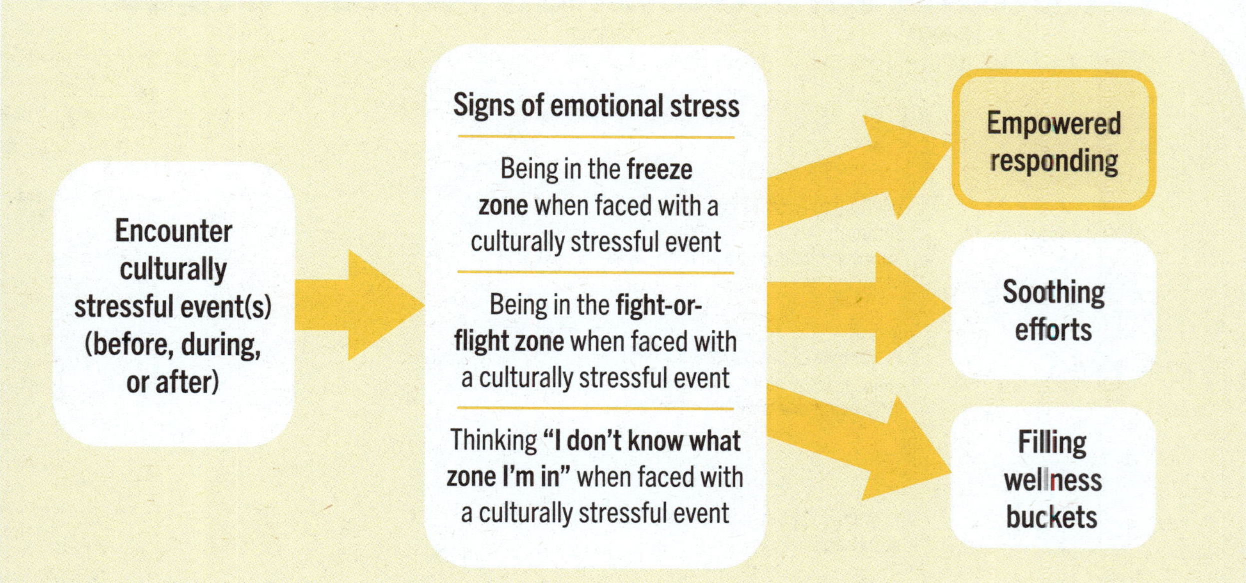

STEPS FOR PRACTICING EMPOWERED RESPONDING

Culturally stressful events may lead to unhelpful action urges, as you learned in Chapter 4. The skill of empowered responding is designed to give you a more helpful alternative (if needed) that you can call up quickly when emotional pain is triggered.

Here are the steps to planning for empowered responding:

1. **Notice your action urges.** The chart My Experiences in Emotional Stress Zones in Chapter 4 (page 66) introduced you to action urges you may have felt when confronted with culturally stressful events. Taking this further, you can begin exploring what empowered responding means for you by understanding which action urges are connected with which emotions. The Emotions and Common Action Urges chart on the next page describes action urges that are commonly experienced when having each emotion.

Pause and Reflect on Your Action Urges

Before moving forward in this chapter, review the **Emotions and Common Action Urges chart** to see if you can write down some of your strongest action urges when faced with culturally stressful events. To practice empowered responding, it's also helpful to know if your action urges are connected with more than one emotion, so list your action urges beside all the emotions they are connected with.

Emotions and Common Action Urges

EMOTION	EXAMPLES OF ACTION URGE(S)	MY ACTION URGE(S)
"I feel anxious."	Wanting to leave or not enter a situation; wanting to get more information about a situation	
"I feel sad."	Wanting to separate from others; wanting to be alone; wanting to stop doing what is enjoyable	
"I feel angry."	Wanting to physically or verbally attack someone or something	
"I feel guilt."	Wanting to hide, confess, apologize, or fix a situation	
"I feel shame."	Wanting to hide, become invisible, or avoid attention	
"I feel hopeless."	Wanting to give up; not wanting to take any action; wanting to minimize effort or energy	
"I feel content."	Wanting to remain consistent with daily activities	
"I feel ____________."		
"I feel ____________."		

2. Brainstorm alternate responses. Sometimes our initial action urges are all we can think about. The emotions connected to these urges can be so strong that it's difficult to seriously consider any alternate coping response. Yet sometimes your best and most empowered option for coping with emotional stress is to engage in a different action than what your urge is telling you to do. Empowered responding can mean choosing to take a step back before moving forward. Or it's choosing to move more slowly rather than frantically racing around.

Pause and Reflect on Alternate Responses

Review the Brainstorming Alternate Responses chart on page 86 and brainstorm some examples of alternate actions you could consider whenever you experience any of these emotions in response to cultural stress.

3. Evaluate your options for responding. Reacting to emotions typically means someone acts on their first initial urge without taking the time to consider any alternate responses. Empowered responding instead encourages us to choose to act on the urges that are most helpful both in the moment and beyond. This can be an extremely tough task. It takes a lot of mental energy to recognize an urge and then determine whether to act on it or not. Yet it's worth learning this skill, because acting on certain urges may lead to unwanted consequences that can place us at a greater risk for further emotional stress. Often, the most empowering response is to choose actions that offer relief from discomfort while also minimizing the likelihood of any unwanted consequences from the actions we've chosen. In this chapter, you will evaluate what could be helpful and unhelpful about the response options you are considering.

4. Create an empowered response plan. Once you've weighed the pros and cons it's time to decide what actions feel best for the situation you're in. This step involves using the worksheet on page 91 to summarize your empowered response and why you chose it.

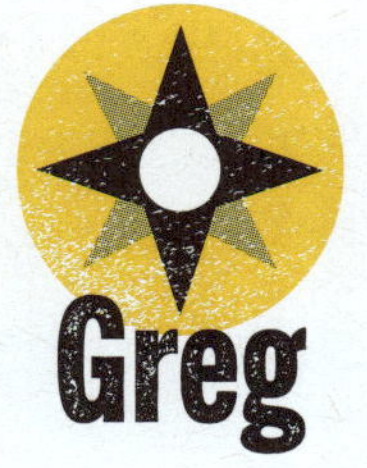

Greg's Empowered Responding

You read in Chapter 4 that Greg was teased and judged by his classmates for wanting to participate in one of his favorite classes. Greg's emotional stress included anger, tension in his hands, and warming throughout his body. These body sensations and emotions caused Greg to have strong action urges to yell at his classmates and say, "Y'all are just mad cuz y'all are too dumb to even know what's going on." See on page 87 how Greg used the steps in this chapter to determine his response to feeling anger.

Brainstorming Alternate Responses

EMOTION	EXAMPLES OF ALTERNATE ACTION URGE(S)	ALTERNATE ACTION(S) I MIGHT CONSIDER
"I feel anxious."	Entering and staying in a situation; not seeking additional information	
"I feel sad."	Seeking social support and connection; maintaining contact with trusted loved ones; investing time and energy in activities that have previously brought enjoyment	
"I feel angry."	Using an activity to calm down; not addressing the situation immediately; not quickly communicating anger until feeling more calm	
"I feel guilt."	Apologize in a meaningful way; change actions to show learning from mistakes	
"I feel shame."	Showcasing, sharing, or highlighting what was previously concealed or hidden	
"I feel hopeless."	Investing time into activities that remain important; taking action to improve circumstances	
"I feel content."	Choosing to stretch outside of comfort zone; trying something new or challenging	
"I feel ____________."		
"I feel ____________."		

1. Notice your action urges. You can see in Greg's BEAT diagram (page 57) that it captures Greg's experience with anger.

When I get angry, I feel like going into attack mode. Nothing physical. I tend to want to run my mouth and let them know what's really on my mind.

2. Brainstorm alternate responses. The level of anger Greg felt after being teased by his peers caused him to focus on finding a way to show his peers that "Enough is enough. I am not taking this anymore." However, he wanted to consider alternate ways of achieving this goal without going into "attack mode."

I guess I could wait a few minutes before saying what's on my mind. Possibly even talk things over with a few friends or one of my closest teachers after class.

3. Evaluate your options for responding. To help him evaluate his options, Greg used the worksheet below. First, he listed the action urge he felt most compelled to act on in that moment. Next, he listed the reasons his action urge may or may not be helpful—specifically thinking of the desired and undesired outcomes that could result from acting on this urge. Finally, he listed an alternate response that he was willing to consider and then similarly evaluated what was most and least helpful about choosing this response.

OPTION	WHAT IS *MOST HELPFUL* ABOUT THE RESPONSE	WHAT IS *LEAST HELPFUL* ABOUT THE RESPONSE
MY INITIAL ACTION URGE: Yell at them	- I make sure they know I don't appreciate being teased or talked about in that way. - I feel proud that I didn't let them walk all over me.	- They might yell back and start a class disruption. - These peers are known to become physically aggressive. - My teacher may not have heard their comments and only think I am yelling without reason. - I may get dismissed from class or an in-school detention.
AN ALTERNATE RESPONSE: Wait until after class and talk it over with my friends	- I can calm down before choosing how I want to respond. - My friends may have some other ideas about how I can handle this. - I can find a response that minimizes the chances I get in trouble.	- I might miss my moment to stand up to them. - I might lose the motivation to stand up to them. - They will think they can keep talking to me in that way.

4. Create an empowered response plan. As shown below, Greg realized that the possibility of being dismissed from class and receiving in-school suspension was too great a risk. He still plans to find a way to communicate to his classmates that "enough is enough," but he ultimately decided that yelling at them in the way he initially felt urged to do was not in his best interest. Importantly, Greg's use of the empowered responding skill demonstrates that there are times when you will realize that it's in your best interest to resist and choose an alternate response to your initial action urges. However, there will also be times when your initial action urges (or at least some version of them) are actually okay to move forward with. This can especially be true if you prioritize regularly practicing this empowered responding skill. Doing so will help you get more familiar with your emotions and learn which action responses are most helpful and empowering—even when facing unimaginable emotional stress.

The response I hope to practice in the moment is:	Wait until after class and talk it over with my friends
My hope is that this response will help me achieve these goals:	Let off steam by talking to my friends and getting their feedback on how to respond moving forward
My hope is that this response will minimize the following unwanted outcomes in the future:	Getting dismissed from class or suspended

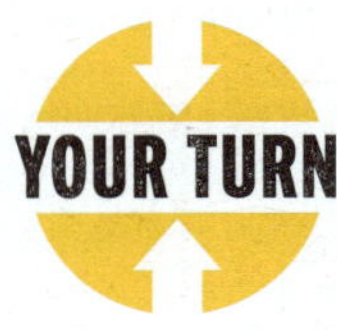

Use the following steps to help you begin thinking about the types of decisions you hope to make when experiencing emotional stress before, during, or after facing a culturally stressful event. To get started, describe a culturally stressful event that has caused you to experience emotional stress.

1. Notice your action urge. Describe any strong action urges you are having (or might have).

Power Up! Tips for Boosting Your Empowered Coping
If you are having difficulty with this step of the empowered responding skill, look back at the action urges listed in the table on page 84.

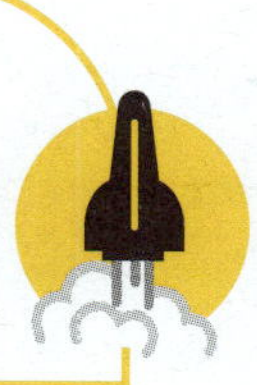

2. **Brainstorm alternate responses.** Describe an alternate action you are willing to consider.

Power Up! Tips for Boosting Your Empowered Coping
If you are having difficulty with this empowered responding skill, look back at the alternate responses listed in the table on page 86.

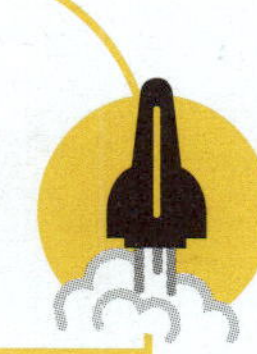

3. **Evaluate your options for responding.** While using the **Evaluating My Responses When Emotionally Stressed worksheet** on page 90 to evaluate your options, consider the following questions:
    - What do you hope to achieve or accomplish in the **short term** with your action responses? How would either response help or not help you achieve this short-term outcome?
    - What do you hope to still be able to achieve or accomplish in the **long term** after this moment passes? Describe how either response would (or would not) give you a chance to still achieve any desired long-term outcomes.
    - Are there any **unwanted outcomes** that could result from either response?
4. **Create your empowered response plan.** Use the **My Empowered Response Plan worksheet** on page 91 to create your action plan for being in the heat of moment during a culturally stressful event.

Evaluating My Responses When Emotionally Stressed

OPTION	WHAT IS *MOST HELPFUL* ABOUT THE RESPONSE	WHAT IS *LEAST HELPFUL* ABOUT THE RESPONSE
MY INITIAL ACTION URGE:		
AN ALTERNATE RESPONSE:		

My Empowered Response Plan

The response I hope to practice in the moment is:	
My hope is that this action will help me achieve these goals:	
My hope is that this action will minimize these unwanted outcomes in the future:	

Chapter 7: Recap and Reflect

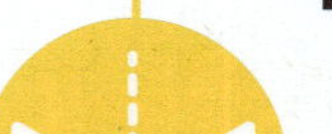

RECAP

- **Empowered responding** is a coping skill that helps you carefully choose which action urges are most or least helpful to act on when feeling emotional stress.
- The steps for practicing the empowered responding skill include:
    1. Notice your action urge.
    2. Consider an alternate response.
    3. Evaluate your options for responding.
    4. Create your empowered response plan.

REFLECT

Hopefully, you have had an opportunity to practice using empowered responding. Before moving forward, take a moment to think about what you learned about empowered responding during your practice and how you hope to use this skill to cope with emotional stress. To do so, answer the questions below.

Calling in your workbook navigators: You may also find it helpful to review your answers to these questions with your workbook navigators, as you may learn which initial action urges they have experienced, get feedback on the reasons they did or did not choose to act on their initial action urges, and learn about alternative responses that helped them in the moment and beyond!

When coping with emotional stress, which action urges have the greatest potential to get in the way of your goals or lead to outcomes that you might feel unhappy with?

When coping with emotional stress, which action urges have the greatest potential to help you achieve your goals and lead to outcomes you can be proud of?

When you evaluate your initial action urges and alternate responses, how have you gone about deciding which action is the best fit for the moment you are in? Do you ever use the *values* from your Who Am I? diagram (page 14) to help you decide how you want to respond to culturally stressful events?

8 How Can I Soothe My Emotional Stress?

While experiencing emotional stress, you may feel stuck trying to answer the question "What can I do to calm myself?" As discussed in Chapter 7, you may be tempted to resolve this challenging dilemma by giving in to action urges that ultimately result in more emotional discomfort and unwanted consequences that you have to manage in the future. In this chapter, you'll learn about **soothing efforts** you can engage in to ride the wave during moments of intense emotional stress.

Specifically, this chapter will feature introductions to:

- *Body-focused coping activities* that may relieve some of the built-up stress and tension within your body
- *Calming activities* that offer a brief distraction and slight relief from the intensity of your emotional discomfort
- Reminders to *seek social support* in ways that help you feel heard and supported

As you review the coping skills throughout this chapter, please keep in mind that they don't represent a complete list of options for soothing your emotions.

Calling in your workbook navigators: Always consider using your workbook navigators to help you brainstorm soothing efforts beyond what is featured in this chapter.

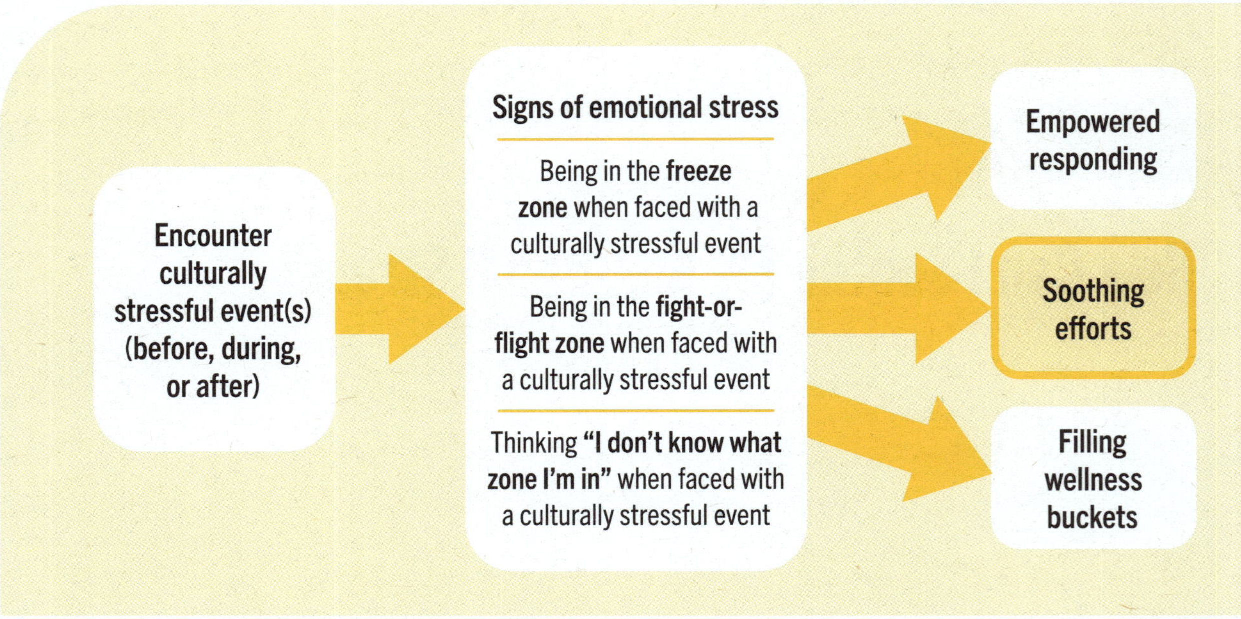

STEPS FOR SOOTHING YOUR UNCOMFORTABLE EMOTIONS

Here are three steps to take to soothe your uncomfortable emotions.

1. Clarify your "riding the wave" expectations. The goal of this chapter is for you to learn to ride the wave of emotional stress by selecting soothing efforts that help you stay afloat as you navigate the uncomfortable and intense waters of your emotions. And, when you do this, it's important to have realistic expectations about what healthy soothing efforts can truly achieve. It's unlikely that any healthy soothing effort will quickly rid you of any uncomfortable body sensations or emotions. Rather, step 1 reminds you to choose to engage in healthy soothing efforts that provide some relief in ways that do not lead to any unwanted problems or consequences for moving forward.

2. Brainstorm soothing efforts. Just as you brainstormed possible alternate responses in Chapter 7, you can brainstorm soothing efforts to help you ride the wave of emotional stress. These soothing efforts offer your mind and body a way to begin the process of relieving some of your built-up stress and discomfort. The following table offers a few prompts to support your brainstorming about the three types of soothing efforts listed at the beginning of the chapter. Also, on the next few pages you'll find tip sheets that offer a few examples of each soothing effort.

Type of soothing effort	Reflection prompt
Body-focused coping	• What options do you have for soothing or relaxing parts of your body? • What options do you have for helping you to temporarily distract from your body sensations until they calm?
Calming activities	• What activities can you engage in that may provide some relief as you ride the wave of emotional stress? • What activities can you engage in that may offer a temporary distraction from your uncomfortable emotions?
Seeking social support	• Are there any trusted family, friends, or authority figures you can spend time with or talk to about your emotional stress? • Even if you are hesitant to reach out to someone, how might you know that you will benefit from seeking social connection as you heal?

3. **Create a plan for practicing your soothing efforts.** List at least three soothing efforts you are willing to practice over the next week. To help you discover the soothing efforts that are most helpful for you when experiencing emotional stress, make sure to practice these efforts *before* you experience emotional stress. Think of your practice as a muscle that you have to exercise so that it becomes conditioned and strengthened for the moment the muscle is truly needed. To find what works best for you, practice your soothing efforts for a few minutes over the next few weeks. And, as you get more familiar and comfortable with the activities you practice, decide which soothing efforts you will try to use when experiencing emotional stress.

TIP SHEETS FOR SOOTHING EFFORTS

Tip Sheet: Building My Body-Focused Coping

Following are a few activities that can help you gradually soothe and release the stress built up in your body. The top three activities (controlled breathing, body scan, and progressive muscle relaxation) all encourage you to ride the wave by turning your attention inward and intentionally focusing on different sensations within your body. However, for some, turning their attention inward when experiencing emotional stress can trigger more discomfort. Sometimes cultural stress can cause us to feel uncomfortable focusing so heavily on our body's sensations for extended periods of time. In such instances, consider engaging in activities that help you to ride the wave by turning your attention outward. You can intentionally focus on the details of your surroundings (grounding: 5-4-3-2-1) or on completing an exercise routine (short-burst exercise). Regardless of which body-focused activity you try, remember these activities are not a magic wand that will immediately make your body's discomfort go away—actually it is likely that your emotional stress will continue to linger even after you practice these activities. Rather, these activities can help you accept and embrace the body discomfort you are feeling while providing some relief from (or at least some release of) stress as you ride the wave.

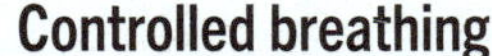

Body scanning

Progressive muscle relaxation

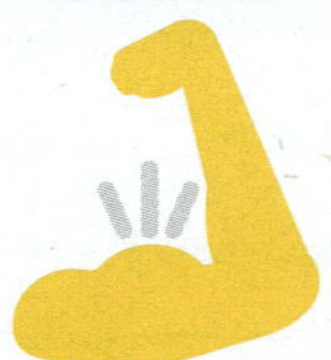

Grounding: 5-4-3-2-1

Short-burst exercise

Create your own

SKILL	WHAT IS THIS SKILL?	HOW TO PRACTICE THIS SKILL
CONTROLLED BREATHING	This skill encourages you to find a breathing pattern that invites your body to begin the process of resting and relaxing. Controlled breathing is not an immediate fix for discomfort, but it is often a good first step toward helping your body begin to relax as you "ride the wave" of emotional stress.	1. Bring your attention to your breath—noticing the rise and fall of your chest. 2. Next, try to prioritize inhaling through your nose and exhaling through your mouth. 3. There is no perfect breathing pattern. Try to find a slow and steady pace of breathing that works for you. Possibly, consider using a breathing pattern where you exhale longer than you inhale. 4. Start by practicing your controlled breathing in short intervals—30, 60, or 90 seconds. 5. If your mind wanders as you practice, try to refocus your attention on the rise and fall of your stomach or chest with each breath.

SKILL	WHAT IS THIS SKILL?	HOW TO PRACTICE THIS SKILL
BODY SCANNING	This skill encourages you to use mindfulness and self-compassion to "ride the wave" of emotional stress. Body scanning is not intended to change the state of the body. Rather, it encourages you to *notice, embrace, and accept* the state of your body. Sometimes the most empowering response to the body is to accept its sensations instead of frantically searching to quickly fix or relieve the sensations.	1. Sit or lie down in a comfortable position. 2. Follow the instructions for controlled breathing. 3. Next, allow your attention to focus on each part of your body for 30–60 seconds. 4. Notice and describe the sensations felt for each body part—possibly noting if a body part feels relaxed or tense, light or heavy. 5. Make efforts to maintain openness and acceptance toward whatever body sensations you feel—saying "I accept and welcome my body in whatever state that it is in.'
PROGRESSIVE MUSCLE RELAXATION (PMR)	This skill encourages you to tense and then slowly release tension in different muscles while maintaining controlled breathing. Practice tensing one muscle group at a time for 15 seconds and then notice how the sensation in that muscle group changes as you release this tension after the 15 seconds. Start by practicing two PMR exercises: (1) focus on your shoulder and neck muscles; and (2) focus on your arm and hand muscles.	1. Find a comfortable seated position. 2. Begin by following instructions for controlled breathing. 3. Tensing: • For shoulders and neck: While sitting upright, slowly bring your shoulders toward your ears and hold them there for 15 seconds. • For arm and hand: While sitting upright, rest the back of your hand on your knee with your palm facing the ceiling, then slowly make a fist for 15 seconds with the back of your hand still resting on your knee. 4. While holding this tension and keeping a controlled breath, notice all the places you feel tension. 5. Try to think to yourself "I accept and welcome the tension in my body." 6. After tensing each muscle group for 15 seconds, gradually release your tensed muscles (slowly lower your shoulders or unclench your fists) and notice the sensations change in your muscle. 7. And, as you notice these changing sensations, think to yourself, "I accept and welcome the relaxing of my body."

√TIP SHEET

SKILL	WHAT IS THIS SKILL?	HOW TO PRACTICE THIS SKILL
GROUNDING: 5-4-3-2-1	This exercise encourages you to shift your attention away from your body and to use your mindfulness skills to observe and describe your surroundings. This can be helpful if attending to your body feels overwhelming or if you want to mix it up—shifting between focusing on your body's sensations with controlled breathing or body scan and focusing on your surroundings. When using this skill, take your time with each observation. Try to discover details about your surroundings that you may not have previously noticed.	1. Notice 5 parts of your surroundings that you can "see." 2. Notice 4 parts of your surroundings that you can "touch." 3. Notice 3 parts of your surroundings that you can "hear." 4. Notice 2 parts of your surroundings that you can "smell." 5. Notice 1 edible part of your surroundings that you can "taste."
SHORT-BURST EXERCISE	Sometimes our bodies need an outlet to release some of the built-up stress. Like a way to burn off some steam. Intense (and if time is limited, short-lasting) exercise can be a useful option for helping your body relieve some stress in a way that is supportive of your overall physical wellness.	1. Choose an exercise activity, such as push-ups, running in place or jogging, walking stairs or a short distance outside, jumping jacks, or weightlifting. 2. Engage in the exercise activity for short intervals and try to anchor your attention to some part of the exercise routine—possibly focusing on engaging in an appropriate exercise technique or counting exercise repetitions. 3. Note: Consult with a medical professional if you are ever concerned that an exercise activity may not be appropriate for you.
CREATE YOUR OWN	What are some other body-focused activities that you can try when experiencing emotional stress?	

Calling in your workbook navigators: Consider asking others what they do to "ride the wave" of their uncomfortable body sensations.

Tip Sheet: Finding Calming Activities

While body-focused activities are primarily about coping with uncomfortable body sensations, think of calming activities as any other activity or task that can provide some relief from (or at least some release of) stress as you ride the wave. Such activities are intended to offer momentary distraction and a helpful alternative to any unhelpful action urges you might have. Calming activities can be used in the heat of the moment when the intensity of emotional stress is rising or lasting longer than desired and can become an activity to focus on while you try to cope with the discomfort you are feeling.

Take a look at the following lists and *circle or highlight* any of the options that appeal to you as potentially calming. Add any others that occur to you.

My Calming Activities

COMFORT	SPIRITUALITY	NATURE	PHYSICAL ACTIVITY
• Lying in a bubble bath • Holding or squeezing a stuffed animal • Listening to upbeat or soothing music • Using favorite scented hand lotion • Burning favorite scented candle • Using favorite scented shampoo or shower gel while bathing • Taking a warm shower • Eating comfort food	• Extending love and kindness to self and others • Completing a devotional reading • Reading a religious text • Praying to a higher power • Giving thanks and acknowledging blessings • Talking to (or seeking guidance from) ancestors • Listening to religious or worship music	• Going on a nature walk • Listening to outdoor sounds • Gardening • Bird watching • Smelling or looking at flowers • Going for a hike • Hosting or attending a cookout	• Playing sports • Playing with or walking a pet • Cleaning or organizing a space • Stretching • Practicing yoga • Going to the gym • Jogging

LEARNING/INSPIRATION	CREATIVITY	FUN	CREATE YOUR OWN
• Looking at old photos • Listening to inspirational podcasts • Reading a good book • Meditating • Starting a crossword puzzle or word search • Journaling • Listening to an audio book	• Cooking • Crocheting or knitting • Painting or drawing • Taking photos • Writing poetry or song lyrics • Building Lego • Making jewelry • Making or playing music	• Playing a game • Watching sports • Trying on clothing • Watching funny video clips • Having a dance party • Watching favorite TV shows • Listening to funny podcasts	(What are some other calming activities that you can try when experiencing emotional stress?)

Tip Sheet: Knowing When to Seek Social Support

Knowing who we can talk to is sometimes not enough to encourage us to seek social support when experiencing emotional stress. Sometimes we may struggle to recall the benefits of sharing vulnerable details about ourselves with others—possibly questioning "How can they even help?" Other times we know that the impacts from cultural stress are heavy and we prefer not to pass along our uncomfortable emotions to others—"I don't want to be a burden." So, to help reduce the obstacles created by these thoughts, take some time to reflect on when seeking support may help you ride the wave of emotional stress. Following are a few reasons that some people may look for support.

Place a check mark next to any of the reasons you may want to challenge yourself to seek support from at least one person in your life. Then take a look at your My Relationship and Community Map (page 33) to identify the people within your social circles you'd be willing to go to when you notice the reasons you checked.

My Reasons for Seeking Social Support

☐ **Overwhelming emotions:** When it gets to the point where it's too overwhelming to handle alone and I need support

☐ **Unsure what I just experienced:** When I just had an uncomfortable experience and I am struggling to make sense of what happened or why it happened

☐ **Unsure how to cope:** When I feel overwhelmed and my usual coping strategies aren't helpful

☐ **Problem solving:** When I want guidance or feedback on how to approach challenging situations, or want to learn how others handled or approached a situation

TIP SHEET

- ☐ **Being self-invalidating:** When I find myself invalidating myself (or telling myself that my feelings don't matter)
- ☐ **Validation:** When I need or want validation (or want someone to show they understand my emotions)
- ☐ **Being self-blaming:** When I find myself blaming myself for what happened
- ☐ **Talking usually helps:** When I know that talking to others typically makes me feel better and helps me feel connected
- ☐ **Feeling alone:** I feel as if I am the only one dealing with these types of stressful experiences
- ☐ **Wanting joy and connection:** It has been a while since I have connected with someone who experiences pride and joy being from my cultural background
- ☐ **Mental health decline:** When I notice my current mental health is on the decline and I'm not doing as well as usual
- ☐ **Being dismissive:** When I notice that I've been dismissing my emotions as not important
- ☐ **Social skill practice:** It doesn't hurt to practice social interactions, and it can allow for deeper connections
- ☐ Other: ______________________
- ☐ Other: ______________________
- ☐ Other: ______________________

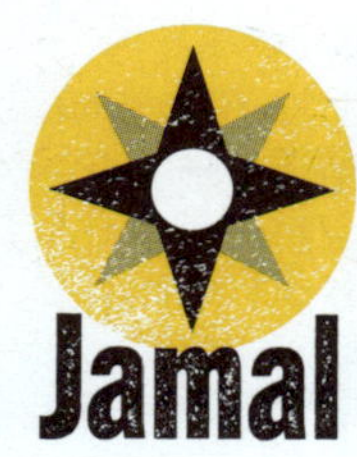

Jamal's Plan for Soothing His Uncomfortable Emotions

Let's revisit Jamal's feelings of sadness, exhaustion, and hopelessness at the end of a typical yet stressful Monday at his office. For a refresher, check out the story in Chapter 3. Following a long day at the office, Jamal noticed that the exhaustion and feelings of hopelessness he felt that night were more familiar than he had previously realized—he had, in fact, been feeling this way for quite some time. Remember, our snapshot of Jamal is occurring just after he has returned home from work. So, as he sits on his couch with this heightened awareness of emotional stress, he is using the steps in this chapter to help him think of ways to soothe the uncomfortable body sensations and emotions he is experiencing.

1. **Clarify your "riding the wave" expectations.** Importantly, by answering "yes" on the next page, Jamal was reminded that riding the wave in the way this chapter encourages meant that he would need to resist engaging in several of his less healthy options for trying to soothe his emotions. For example, Jamal has used alcohol and escaping into video games until the early hours of the morning to soothe his emotions. But, as you might guess, these efforts can actually backfire in the long run if used repeatedly. Instead, he is trying to maintain the mindset "I want to find a soothing effort that helps me now without causing problems for me later."

WHAT TO THINK ABOUT	RESPONSE
Riding the wave expectations *What body sensations or emotions are you seeking relief from?*	Physically tired Feeling sad and hopeless
Have you reminded yourself that your soothing efforts may not quickly or immediately get rid of your emotional stress?	● Yes ○ No

2. Brainstorm soothing efforts. Jamal used the reflection prompts to help him brainstorm options for each type of soothing effort. Of note, some of the options he thought of ultimately were not healthy ways to ride the wave. But he didn't stop there. He kept brainstorming. You might also feel tempted to give in to action urges that are not the most helpful in the long term. That's okay. Just keep the brainstorming process going until you think of soothing efforts that aren't likely to cause more emotional stress after the uncomfortable situation has passed.

WHAT TO THINK ABOUT	RESPONSE
Body-focused coping *What options do you have for soothing or relaxing parts of your body?* *What options do you have for helping you temporarily distract from your body sensations until they calm?*	I could exercise right now, but I'm so tired. I guess I could try that grounding activity on the tip sheet. I kind of don't want to focus on how tired I am right now.
Calming activities *What activities can you engage in that may provide some relief as you "ride the wave" of emotional stress?* *What activities can you engage in that may offer a temporary distraction from your uncomfortable emotions?*	I really want to just drink a few and play video games, but I guess I could cook a quick meal and take my mind off things by watching one of my favorite shows.
Seek social support *Are there any trusted family, friends, or authority figures you can spend time with or talk with about your emotional stress?* *Even if you are hesitant to reach out to someone, how might you know that you will benefit from seeking social connection as you heal?*	It's kind of late, but maybe I could text one of my former classmates who also just started a new job. Maybe she'll be down to chat today or sometime this week.

3. Create a plan for practicing your soothing efforts. After brainstorming different soothing efforts, Jamal decided how he wanted to seek relief after work. And, beyond this moment he is in, Jamal also thought of ways to continue practicing his soothing efforts—possibly even building a routine for proactively practicing this skill rather than waiting until the peak of his emotional stress to use the skill.

SOOTHING EFFORT	WHEN DO YOU WANT TO PRACTICE?
1. Grounding: 5-4-3-2-1	I want to try this tonight for sure. But it also might be helpful when I go back to office.
2. Cooking a meal	I really enjoy cooking new things. Maybe I can try to cook at least two new meals a week. The meal planning, cooking, and eating might give my mind something else to focus on for a bit.
3. Text my friend	I have been told I have a tendency to suffer in silence. Maybe it would be good to schedule at least one check-in call with a friend per week.

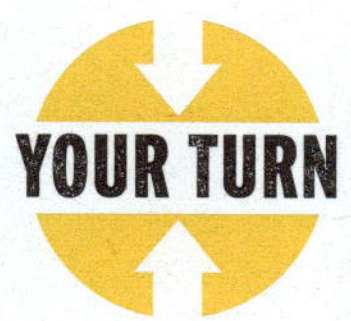

Use the steps below to help you find the soothing efforts that you can use to help you "ride the wave" when experiencing emotional stress.

1. **Clarify your riding the wave expectations.** Use the prompts in the worksheet below to help focus your "riding the wave" expectations.

2. **Brainstorm soothing efforts.** Try to brainstorm at least three options for each category in the worksheet on page 104.

My Riding the Wave Expectations

WHAT TO THINK ABOUT	MY RESPONSE
Riding the wave expectations *What body sensations or emotions are you seeking relief from?*	
Have you reminded yourself that your soothing efforts may not quickly or immediately get rid of your emotional stress?	○ Yes ○ No

My Toolkit of Soothing Efforts

WHAT TO THINK ABOUT	RESPONSE
Body-focused coping What are the top three body-focused activities you could engage in to ride the wave of intense bodily sensations?	**1.** **2.** **3.**
Calming activities What are the top three calming activities you can engage in to soothe your mind and emotions?	**1.** **2.** **3.**
Seeking social support What are the top three signs that you might benefit from seeking emotional support from your support system?	**1.** **2.** **3.**
Other soothing efforts What other soothing efforts might be helpful for you to try when experiencing emotional stress?	**1.** **2.** **3.**

Power Up! Tips for Boosting Your Empowered Coping

Keep a list. When we are emotionally stressed, our brains have a way of forgetting many of the coping options we have available to us. In addition to the tip sheets on pages 95–101, consider keeping a list of soothing efforts that helped you in the past. Possibly, list these efforts in your phone, on your bathroom mirror, or on notecards so you can quickly reference and use for brainstorming.

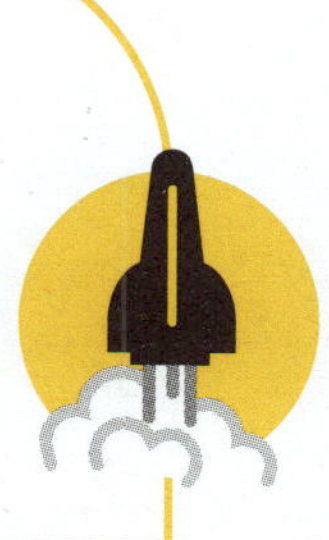

3. Create a plan for practicing your soothing efforts. Now, it's time to choose a few soothing efforts to put into practice (below).

My Plan for Practicing Soothing Efforts

Instructions: List at least three soothing efforts you are willing to practice over the next week and then set specific goals for when you will practice each effort before deciding if this is a soothing effort you want to add to your empowered coping toolkit.

SOOTHING EFFORT	WHEN DO YOU WANT TO PRACTICE?
1.	
2.	
3.	

Chapter 8: Recap and Reflect

RECAP

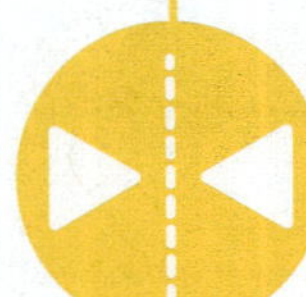

- **Soothing efforts** are options for seeking some relief from uncomfortable body sensations and emotions.
- The steps for practicing the soothing my emotions skill include:
    1. Clarify your "riding the wave" expectations.
    2. Brainstorm soothing efforts.
    3. Create a plan for practicing your soothing efforts.

REFLECT

Hopefully, you have had an opportunity to practice using your soothing efforts. Before moving forward, take a moment to think about what you learned about soothing your emotions during your practice and how you hope to use this skill to cope with emotional stress. To do so, answer the questions below.

Calling in your workbook navigators: You may also find it helpful to review your answers to these questions with your workbook navigators, as you may learn what soothing efforts they have found the most and least helpful. Also, you may find that they are willing to join you as you practice your soothing efforts. It can be nice to have a bit of accountability and support when trying new ways of coping.

What activities best help you *temporarily distract* yourself from the intensity of your emotions?

What activities best help you *relax and soothe* your bodily sensations or emotions?

Do you ever use any of the *strengths* or *interests* from your Who Am I? diagram (page 14) to help you brainstorm your soothing efforts?

9

How Can I Make Healthy Decisions over Time as I Heal from Emotional Stress?

Sometimes emotional stress can make it hard to sustain your healthy daily routines. Finding yourself in the freeze zone (see My Experiences in Emotional Stress Zones on page 66) in particular can trigger urges to give up on important life goals and disconnect from meaningful relationships. You may even limit the time and energy you invest in enjoyable activities that bring you happiness. Using the skill of empowered responding (Chapter 7) to resist these urges can help. But if you struggle for days, weeks, or even months with strong urges to withdraw, the weight of emotional stress may start to interfere much more in your daily life.

This chapter gives you a way to build resilience and promote healing so you can make healthy decisions over time even while healing from emotional pain. It's a coping skill called **filling wellness buckets.** It involves finding ways to maintain daily routines that promote emotional and physical wellness. Think of this coping skill as your way of adding positives to your life while you're also trying to reduce the negatives—like an emotional bank account where you try to maintain a positive emotional balance despite the emotional drain of cultural stress on you. You'll practice continuing to invest time and energy into important areas of your life as emotional healing progresses.

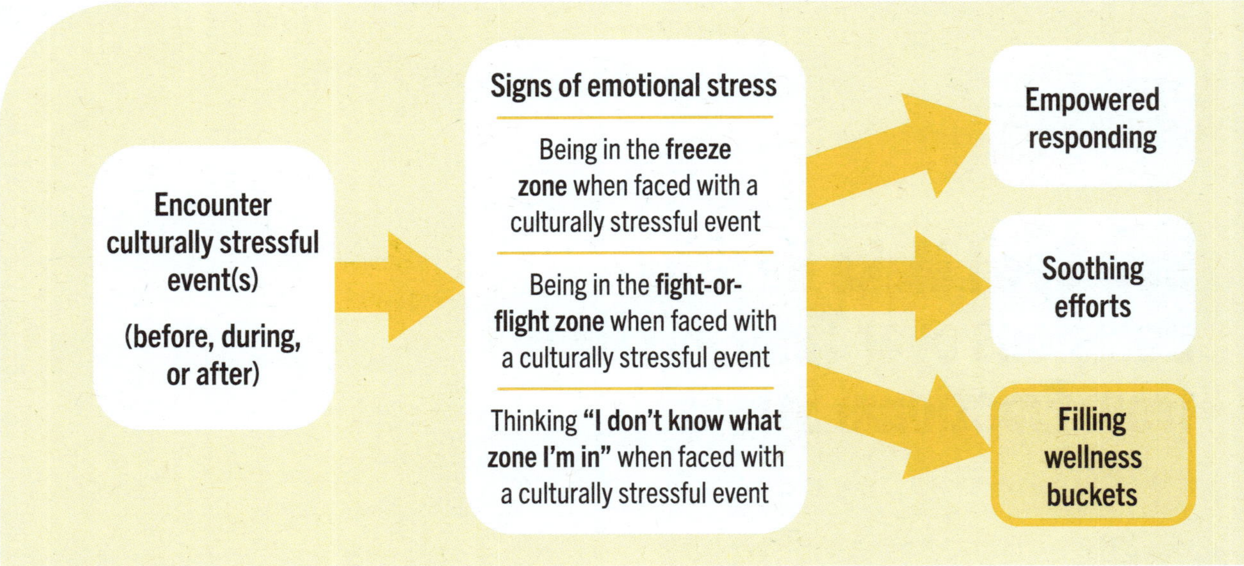

FILL YOUR WELLNESS BUCKETS

This coping skill encourages you to make efforts to regularly invest time and energy in four areas that are important to health and resilience:

- Physical wellness
- Social connection
- Fun and enjoyment
- Accomplishment and mastery

Notice the word *effort* here. Filling your wellness buckets may not always feel great, exciting, or stress relieving. Sometimes an effort will feel like it adds only a tiny drop to a bucket. But it's still important to honor your ability to continuously make efforts to add positive experiences to your life—even when cultural stress remains around you. Taking the time to acknowledge these efforts can remind you what remains within your control and help you think of ways you can still have influence over your life and emotional wellness.

The following steps will get you started.

1. **Clarify which wellness buckets you want to fill.** When you know that you have been emotionally stressed for a few days or weeks at a time, it can be helpful to consider whether any wellness buckets are running particularly low. Remember, the act of filling your wellness buckets includes any efforts you make to invest

time and energy in physical wellness, social connection, fun and enjoyment, or feeling accomplished. So, step 1 is all about asking yourself, "Which buckets have I struggled to make efforts to fill recently?" or "Where have I had difficulty investing my effort and time?"

2. **Brainstorm options for filling your wellness buckets.** Once you have identified the buckets that are running low, it's important to brainstorm ways you can reasonably begin to reinvest time and energy into filling these buckets.

Pause and Reflect on Ways You Might Fill Your Buckets

On page 110 are some options for filling each wellness bucket. *Circle or check* any options that you already do (or even would like to do). Also, this is not an exhaustive list, so please add in your own examples.

3. **Create a wellness plan.** Even though you may be able to brainstorm the routines you want to keep, you might need extra support to follow through on filling your wellness buckets. Emotional stress has a way of interfering with plans to engage in health-boosting activities. To make these activities part of your routine, try scheduling your bucket filling. Look over your weekly calendar and then identify times in your day when you can make an effort to fill each of your wellness buckets. To sustain your motivation, you also might find it helpful to set a goal for each effort at the beginning of the week. For example, you might set a goal for completing an activity/task a certain number of times per week (doing a morning walk and stretching three times per week) or for a certain amount of time (cleaning for at least 30 minutes).

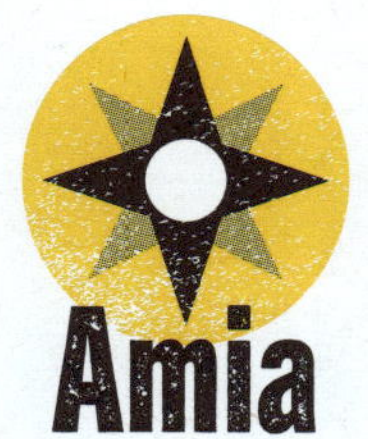

Amia's Plan for Filling Her Wellness Buckets

Amia recently noticed that the emotional stress she experienced from her interactions with a few insensitive classmates had decreased her motivation to go to school so much that she started doing something she never thought she'd do—skipping school. For two weeks, she woke up and left her home as if she was going to school, but instead Amia hung out in the neighborhood around her school until the end of the school day. Eventually, her school contacted her parents to ask why Amia had not attended school for two weeks, which created a whole new source of emotional stress. Amia has also noticed herself wanting to avoid more than just school—she's becoming less and less willing to take public transportation, spend

Options for Filling Wellness Buckets

☐ Physical wellness
- ☐ Prioritizing rest
- ☐ Maintaining good hygiene
- ☐ Keeping a consistent sleep routine
- ☐ Eating consistent/healthy meals
- ☐ Maintaining an exercise routine
- ☐ Seeking medical support when needed
- ☐ Taking medications as prescribed
- ☐ Not relying on unprescribed substances
- ☐ Other: ______________
- ☐ Other: ______________
- ☐ Other: ______________

☐ Social connection
- ☐ Initiating hangouts
- ☐ Accepting invitations to hangout
- ☐ Initiating texts/calls
- ☐ Responding to texts/calls
- ☐ Sharing emotions with loved ones
- ☐ Attending social events
- ☐ Spending time with family and friends
- ☐ Meeting new people
- ☐ Other: ______________
- ☐ Other: ______________
- ☐ Other: ______________

☐ Fun/enjoyment
- ☐ Spending time on hobbies
- ☐ Watching favorite show
- ☐ Completing art project
- ☐ Listening to music or a podcast
- ☐ Eating comfort foods
- ☐ Playing a game
- ☐ Dancing
- ☐ Reading a book or short story
- ☐ Going for a walk or bike ride
- ☐ Trying something new
- ☐ Other: ______________
- ☐ Other: ______________
- ☐ Other: ______________

☐ Accomplished/mastery
- ☐ Checking off something on your to-do list
- ☐ Completing a chore or assignment
- ☐ Learning about something new
- ☐ Practicing a skill
- ☐ Teaching someone else how to do something
- ☐ Helping or supporting someone else or your community
- ☐ Creating, designing, or building something
- ☐ Organizing your schedule
- ☐ Creating a plan for completing a future task
- ☐ Other: ______________
- ☐ Other: ______________
- ☐ Other: ______________

time in public parks, or hang out at her local shopping mall due to concerns of being judged negatively for her racial and cultural background. As you might guess, such a broad impact from emotional stress is weighing heavily on Amia. Let's see how she uses the exercises in this chapter to help her resist these broad avoidance urges.

1. **Clarify which wellness buckets you want to fill.** Using the reflection prompts in the following worksheet, Amia gained clarity about where she needed to invest effort into improving her wellness.

WHAT TO THINK ABOUT	MY RESPONSES
Physical wellness *Have you noticed yourself having any* ***difficulty maintaining any physical or emotional health routines?***	○ Yes ● No ○ Sometimes
Social connection *Have you noticed yourself having any* ***difficulty staying connected with family, friends, and others close to you?***	● Yes ○ No ○ Sometimes
Fun and enjoyment *Have you noticed yourself having any* ***difficulty investing time and energy in activities that typically bring you enjoyment?***	○ Yes ○ No ● Sometimes
Accomplishment and mastery *Have you noticed yourself having any* ***difficulty investing time and energy in completing tasks that typically make you feel proud and accomplished?***	● Yes ○ No ○ Sometimes

2. Brainstorm options for filling your wellness buckets. Amia brainstormed the following ideas for filling her wellness buckets:

PHYSICAL WELLNESS

1. Keeping a 10 p.m. bedtime
2. Morning walk 3x/week
3. Stretching 3x/week
4.
5.

SOCIAL CONNECTION

1. Text friend from mosque
2. Join Sister's Quran class
3. Attend youth group at Islamic Community Center
4.
5.

FUN/ENJOYMENT

1. Listening to music daily
2. Practice singing 2x/week
3. Watch a movie per month
4.
5.

ACCOMPLISHED/MASTERY

1. Attend all my classes daily
2. Complete homework daily
3. Do community service 1x/month
4.
5.

3. Create a wellness plan. Amia created the following plan for a week during her school year.

DAY	PHYSICAL WELLNESS	SOCIAL CONNECTION	FUN/ENJOYMENT	ACCOMPLISHED/ MASTERY
SUNDAY	- Bedtime: 10 p.m.	- Attend Youth Group at Islamic Community Center	- Updating music playlists	- Finish homework for Monday
MONDAY	- Bedtime: 10 p.m. - Morning walk	- Text at least one friend	- Listening to music playlists before and after school	- Attend 7 out of 7 classes - Complete at least 1 hour of homework
TUESDAY	- Bedtime: 10 p.m.	- Text at least one friend	- Listening to music playlists before and after school	- Attend 7 out of 7 classes - Complete at least 1 hour of homework
WEDNESDAY	- Bedtime: 10 p.m. - Morning walk	- Text at least one friend	- Listening to music playlists before and after school	- Attend 7 out of 7 classes - Complete at least 1 hour of homework
THURSDAY	- Bedtime: 10 p.m.		- Listening to music playlists before and after school	- Attend 7 out of 7 classes - Complete at least 1 hour of homework
FRIDAY	- Bedtime: whenever - Morning walk	- Text at least one friend	- Listening to music playlists before and after school	- Attend 7 out of 7 classes
SATURDAY	- Bedtime: whenever	- Attend my Quran class	- Watching a new movie - Practice singing	- Attend my Youth Group's community service event

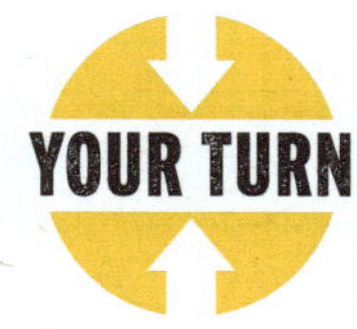

1. Clarify which wellness buckets you want to fill. Use the reflection prompts on the facing page to help you identify which wellness buckets you want to focus on filling in this moment. *Circle or highlight* yes, no, or sometimes for each bucket.

Which of My Wellness Buckets Need to Be Filled?

WHAT TO THINK ABOUT	MY RESPONSES
Physical wellness *Have you noticed yourself having any **difficulty maintaining any physical or emotional health routines?***	o Yes o No o Sometimes
Social connection *Have you noticed yourself having any **difficulty staying connected with family, friends, and others close to you?***	o Yes o No o Sometimes
Fun and enjoyment *Have you noticed yourself having any **difficulty investing time and energy in activities that typically bring you enjoyment?***	o Yes o No o Sometimes
Accomplishment and mastery *Have you noticed yourself having any **difficulty investing time and energy in completing tasks that typically make you feel proud and accomplished?***	o Yes o No o Sometimes

2. **Brainstorm options for filling your wellness buckets.** Referring to the Options for Filling Wellness Buckets list on page 110, think of three to five activities you can regularly do in the coming weeks to fill your (1) physical wellness, (2) social connection, (3) fun/enjoyment, and (4) accomplished/mastery buckets and write them in the worksheet on the next page.

Power Up! Tips for Boosting Your Empowered Coping

Calling in your workbook navigators: This might be a good place to consult your workbook navigators for ideas, especially if you and the navigator often participate in healthy activities together, whether it's taking a morning run in a park, having a potluck dinner, or scheduling game nights with friends or family.

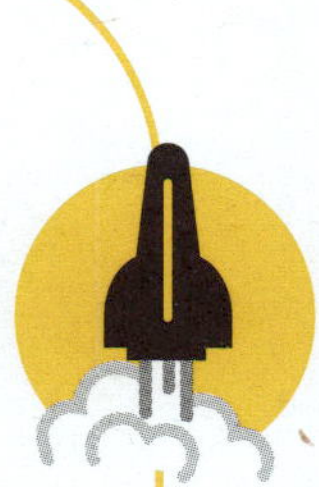

My Wellness Buckets Activities and Tasks

PHYSICAL WELLNESS

1. ______________________________

2. ______________________________

3. ______________________________

4. ______________________________

5. ______________________________

SOCIAL CONNECTION

1. ______________________________

2. ______________________________

3. ______________________________

4. ______________________________

5. ______________________________

FUN/ENJOYMENT

1. ______________________________

2. ______________________________

3. ______________________________

4. ______________________________

5. ______________________________

ACCOMPLISHED/MASTERY

1. ______________________________

2. ______________________________

3. ______________________________

4. ______________________________

5. ______________________________

3. Create a wellness plan. Now create a plan for when and how often you are going to make efforts to fill each of your wellness buckets and enter it into the worksheet below.

My Wellness Plan

DAY	PHYSICAL WELLNESS	SOCIAL CONNECTION	FUN/ ENJOYMENT	ACCOMPLISHED/ MASTERY
SUNDAY				
MONDAY				
TUESDAY				
WEDNESDAY				
THURSDAY				
FRIDAY				
SATURDAY				

Power Up! Tips for Boosting Your Empowered Coping

- **Start small.** If you notice that several buckets are running low, start small. Pick one bucket to focus on per day (or even per week) until you notice yourself more regularly filling this bucket.
- **Set yourself up for success.** Try to start with low-effort activities, such as activities that do not require a lot of planning or time, before scheduling high-effort activities.
- **Find bucket-filling partners.** Sometimes it can be hard to fill these buckets alone. So, consider sharing your wellness plan (step 3) with your workbook navigators (the people you listed on page 6). Possibly, they can join you in completing some of these health-boosting activities, or at least check in with you to see how your bucket filling is going.

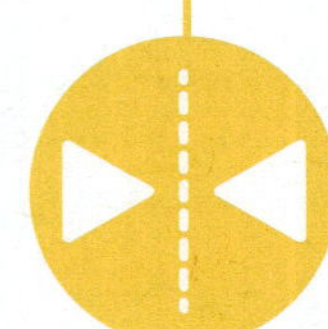

Chapter 9: Recap and Reflect

RECAP

- **Filling wellness buckets** describes continuing to make efforts to invest time in activities or tasks that promote physical wellness, social connection, fun/enjoyment, and accomplishment/mastery.
- The steps for practicing the filling wellness buckets skill include:
  1. Clarify which wellness buckets to focus on.
  2. Brainstorm options for filling your wellness buckets.
  3. Create a wellness plan.

REFLECT

Hopefully you have had an opportunity to practice using your wellness plan. Before moving forward, take a moment to think about what you learned about filling your wellness buckets during your practice and how you hope to use any of these decisions to cope with emotional stress. To do so, answer the upcoming questions.

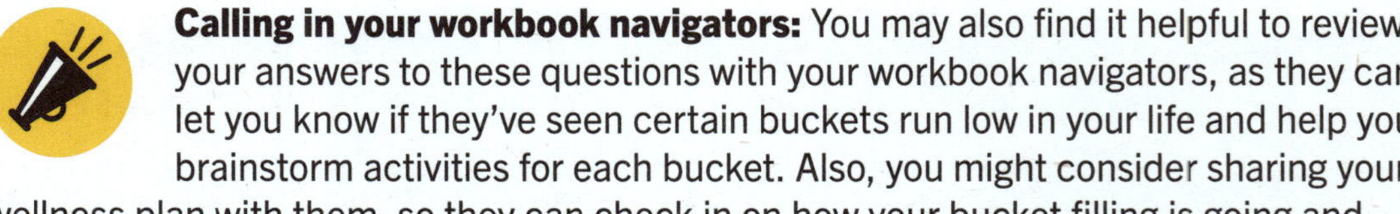

Calling in your workbook navigators: You may also find it helpful to review your answers to these questions with your workbook navigators, as they can let you know if they've seen certain buckets run low in your life and help you brainstorm activities for each bucket. Also, you might consider sharing your wellness plan with them, so they can check in on how your bucket filling is going and celebrate you as you meet your bucket-filling goals.

What are the areas of your life you want to do your best to invest time into while you heal from emotional stress?

What ways have you learned to invest time into your *physical well-being* in your daily life (sleep, meals, exercise)? Or into your *social connections* in your daily life?

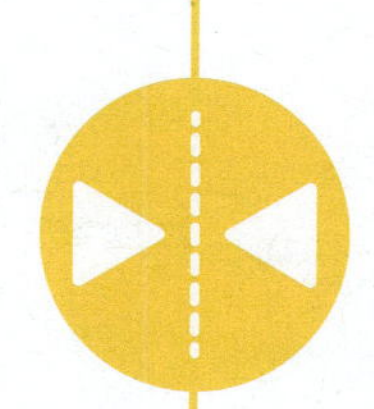

How have you created opportunities to experience *enjoyment/fun* in your daily life? Or opportunities that help you feel *accomplished or masterful?*

PART TWO SUMMARY AND TAKEAWAYS

- **Emotional stress** describes moments when we experience uncomfortable body sensations and emotions from culturally stressful events.
- In Chapter 4 you learned how to notice the moments when you're experiencing emotional stress. You learned to use the BEAT diagram and the emotional stress zones chart to practice **mindfulness.**
- In Chapter 5 you learned that when experiencing emotional stress, you can become critical of and judgmental about your BEAT reactions. To navigate self-criticism, you can learn **self-compassion** to show kindness and understanding toward your emotional stress.
- In Chapter 6 you discovered any **emotional stress coping** skills you brought to this workbook and any coping skills you wanted to strengthen using the processes outlined in Chapters 7, 8, and 9.
- In Chapter 7 you learned that emotional stress can bring on strong urges to engage in unhelpful responses to cultural stress. To navigate these urges, **empowered responding** can help you carefully choose which action urges are most or least helpful to act on when feeling emotional stress.
- In Chapter 8 you learned that emotional stress may take time to reduce and calm. To ride the waves of emotional stress you can use different **soothing efforts** (body-focused coping activities, calming activities, seeking support).
- In Chapter 9 you learned that emotional stress can make it hard to maintain wellness efforts in daily life. **Filling wellness buckets** can help you restore and maintain routines that promote your physical wellness, maintain social connection, provide opportunities to experience fun and enjoyment, and offer opportunities to feel a sense of accomplishment and mastery.

TRACK YOUR EMOTIONAL STRESS COPING

Whenever you notice yourself experiencing emotional stress when facing a culturally stressful event, keep track of the empowered coping skills you use to ride the wave of uncomfortable body sensations and emotions you experience. In the following worksheet, enter the date when you notice emotional stress and then describe whether you used any coping skills from Chapter 5 (**self-compassion**), Chapter 7 (**empowered responding**), Chapter 8 (**soothing efforts**), or Chapter 9 (**filling wellness buckets**). Also, there is a column for any empowered coping decisions you make that do not fall into these four categories.

My Emotional Stress Coping

NOTICED EMOTIONAL STRESS	SELF-COMPASSION	EMPOWERED RESPONDING	SOOTHING EFFORTS	FILLING WELLNESS BUCKETS	OTHER EMOTIONAL STRESS COPING
Date:					
Date:					
Date:					
Date:					
Date:					
Date:					

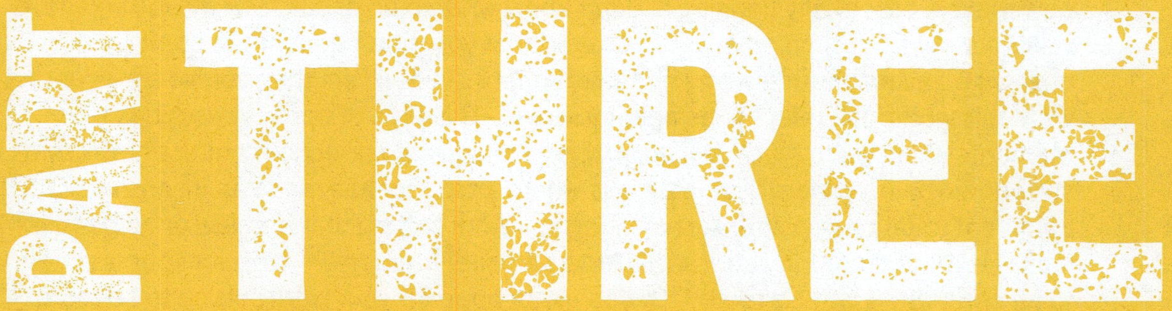

PART THREE

How to Boost Your Sense of Agency and Control

Have you ever been face to face with a culturally stressful event and felt completely powerless—essentially thinking "I don't know what to do or say"? Or maybe you have walked away from such an event frustrated that you didn't do more to confront or challenge any unfair judgments or mistreatment of you. If so, then you've experienced what this workbook refers to as **agency stress.** This type of impact describes the moments when we're stuck *feeling unable to change or correct* our culturally stressful surroundings. Imagine sitting in a class where a teacher has made an insensitive racial comment (relationship stressor) or being in a work setting that had few or no people who look like you (community stressor). Understandably, you might wish for your teacher to be confronted and corrected. Or you might hope for your work setting to be more inclusive and diverse. In either case, agency stress would describe any moments when you might feel upset or discouraged by your inability to make either of these goals a reality.

Part Three explains ways to expand your sense of agency and control within the relationships and community spaces that are your greatest sources of cultural stress. Don't get me wrong. The realities and limitations of cultural stress are still present, and this section of the workbook promises no magic solutions for erasing all culturally stressful events from your life. Rather, *you will enhance your empowered coping by better understanding the moments when you're experiencing agency stress and expanding your definition of what* agency *and* control *can mean within your surroundings.*

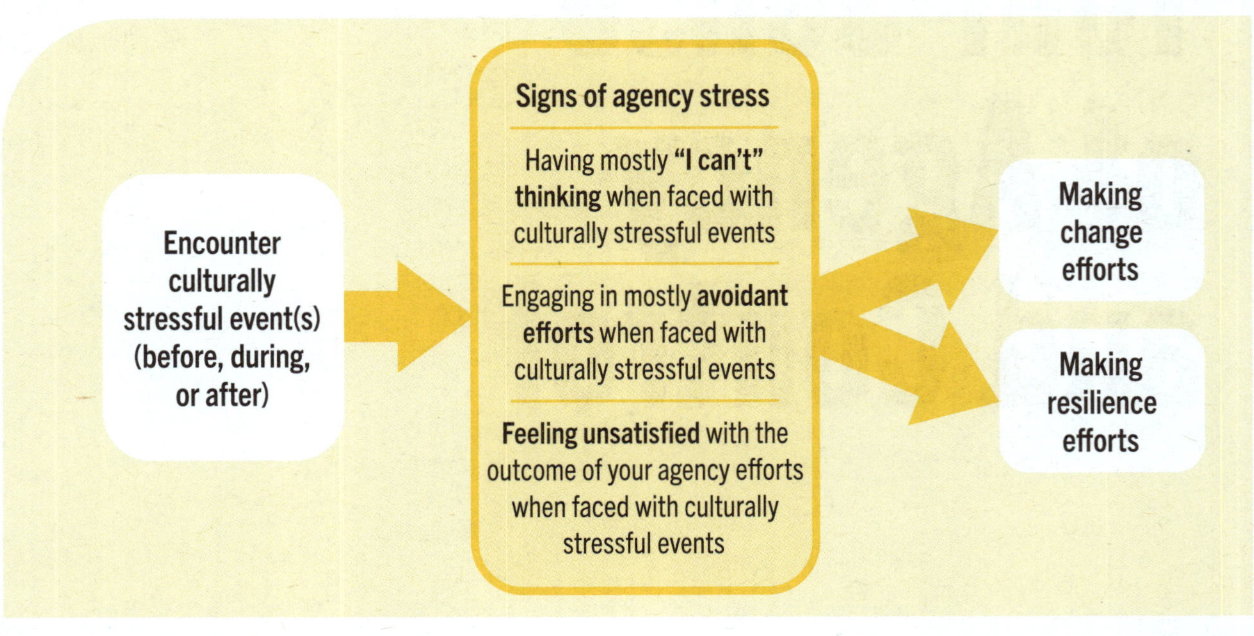

10 Noticing When I Experience Agency Stress

Throughout this workbook, you've used the BEAT diagram (at right) to help you know when and how you are impacted by a culturally stressful event. In this chapter, you'll learn to use the BEAT diagram to help you notice **agency stress.** The exercises in this chapter will help you notice specific details in your action urges and thoughts that suggest you're feeling a lack of control or agency within a relationship or while in a community space.

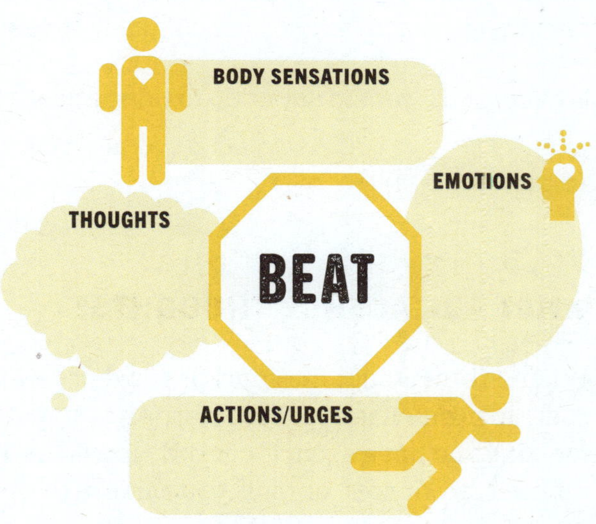

WHAT ARE CHANGE EFFORTS?

Change can be very necessary. It can also be scary, especially when it comes to making social spaces less culturally stressful for POCs. Of course, it's great when politicians, lawyers, teachers, bosses, and even friends make efforts to change culturally stressful spaces in ways that benefit POCs. But often the responsibility for change falls on the shoulders of POCs, meaning that you may feel the pressure to come up with clever or strategic actions to make spaces less stressful for yourself.

Does this pressure sound familiar? Have you ever felt like you wanted to change, correct, or improve your surroundings? One way to notice whether you've had these desires for change is by looking at the action urges in your BEAT diagram any time you're faced with a culturally stressful situation. In such moments you might notice urges to:

- Confront someone and tell them to "stop" their insensitive behavior
- Correct any inaccurate information they have about your background
- Participate in events that seek to improve your community

In this book these actions are called **change efforts.** You'll learn a lot more about change efforts throughout Part Three. For now, just start reflecting on any instances when you've had urges to engage in a change effort.

Pause and Reflect on Your Change Efforts

Take a moment to think about any ways you have wanted to change a relationship or community space that has felt culturally stressful.

What did you want to say or do to bring about change in your surroundings?

WHAT ARE AGENCY THOUGHTS?

When I think about the concept of agency, words like *control, power,* and *influence* come to mind. Each of these words has something in common: an "I can" mindset. To feel like you have agency, control, power, and influence, you must have an idea of the abilities, resources, or tools you *can* use to address the obstacle you're up against.

You've undoubtedly also experienced moments when you lack a strong sense of agency. At those times, you're probably operating with some form of an "I can't" mindset: "I can't do this because I don't know how to solve the problem" or "I can't say that because it will just make things worse." Whenever you notice urges or wishes to engage in a change effort, your "I can" or "I can't" thinking could determine whether those urges ever become actions.

HOW TO DECIDE WHETHER YOU CAN MAKE CHANGES TO LESSEN CULTURAL STRESS

It's not easy to make decisions about how to respond to culturally stressful events in the moment. But you can reflect on past incidents and evaluate why you did or did not feel able to make the change effort that came to mind at that time. When you become practiced at this type of analysis, it becomes easier to notice the presence of an "I can" versus "I can't" mindset as well as how either mindset may influence how you decide to act. Here are the steps.

1. **Identify the change effort you feel an urge to make in response to the culturally stressful event.** These urges often feel somewhat automatic, so it can be helpful to look more closely at them.

2. **Identify any "I can" and "I can't" agency thoughts that come up when considering turning this urge into an action.** Examples of thoughts that fall into three common categories are shown in the following table (a version for you to fill out appears later in the chapter).

3. **Determine whether you feel (or felt) able to engage in the change effort.** Finally, take a moment to consider whether your agency thoughts suggest you mostly do or do not feel able to pursue the change you want in that moment. As we will discuss in detail later, feeling as if you are not able to engage in your change efforts is a sign of what this book calls *agency stress.*

EXPLANATIONS FOR AGENCY THINKING	WHAT TO THINK ABOUT	REASONS "I CAN"	REASONS "I CAN'T"
PERSONAL ABILITIES	Do you feel like you have the skills, traits, or abilities to engage in an effective change effort when faced with a culturally stressful event?	"I can say something because I am quick with my comebacks."	"I can't say anything. I'll just choke and freeze under pressure."
ACCESS TO SUPPORT	Do you feel like you have any support from the people around you to engage in an effective change effort when faced with a culturally stressful event?	"I can say something because I know my boy will back me up."	"Even if I say anything, I'll be alone. No one will have my back."
COSTS VERSUS BENEFITS	Do you feel like the benefits of engaging in a change effort outweigh the costs of not trying to do so?	"I want to say something even if they don't like it. They need to know this isn't right."	"I can't say anything, because if I do I'll probably lose it and get fired."

Jamal

Jamal's Analysis of His Agency Thoughts

Culturally stressful event: Jamal's coworkers sing insensitive lyrics

One day, Jamal walks into the work breakroom and overhears several White coworkers singing the latest rap song. As Jamal walks by them, they nod his way and continue singing the song's hook, which repeats the *N*-word multiple times. This makes Jamal uncomfortable, and he feels an urge to do something about this.

1. What change efforts might you have the urge to make in this scenario? Jamal wrote down an action urge focused on confronting his colleagues in a way that would try to change their insensitive behavior.

I could tell them "Don't sing that in front of me."

2. Use the My Agency Thoughts worksheet to identify reasons you may or may not feel able to engage in these change efforts. From Jamal's responses, we see that he feels like he has the ability to act on this urge but also has some concerns about not being supported or running into unwanted consequences that are making his "I can't" thinking pretty strong in this moment.

EXPLANATIONS FOR AGENCY THINKING	WHAT TO THINK ABOUT	REASONS "I CAN"	REASONS "I CAN'T"
PERSONAL ABILITIES	Do you feel like you have the skills, traits, or abilities to engage in an effective change effort in this situation?	Yes, I could see myself saying that.	
ACCESS TO SUPPORT	Do you feel like you have any support from the people around you to engage in an effective change effort in this situation?		Not sure anyone else in the office would see it from my perspective. They'll probably be like, "What's the big deal? They are just singing the lyrics of a song."
COSTS VERSUS BENEFITS	Do you feel like the benefits of engaging in a change effort would outweigh the costs of not trying to do so in this situation?	The benefits would be that they stop singing.	But I could see them telling people I am too sensitive. Or they might get really weird around me, which would just make my workday more exhausting. Right now, saying something feels more costly than beneficial.

3. Based on your "I can" and "I can't" thinking above, do you feel able to engage in any change effort(s)? It seems that ultimately Jamal concluded "I can't" act on this urge right now. For some, such a conclusion is not bothersome. They make this assessment and just move on without any stressful feelings. However, there are times, as for Jamal in this example, where such "I can't" thinking and choosing not to make a change effort can really eat at you over time. That's agency stress—the moments when you feel stuck wishing and wanting to do or say more to change your culturally stressful surroundings yet you feel that you "can't."

I definitely have the ability to say something and probably should, but I don't really know if it's worth it. Ugh, this decision will probably eat at me for the rest of the day.

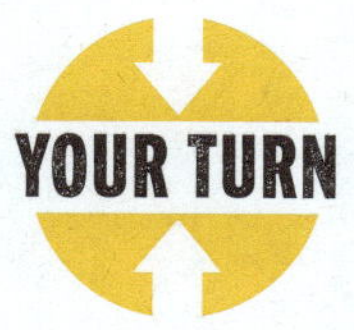

Below is an example of a culturally stressful event. Take a look and see what change efforts naturally come up when you read the scenario. Then use the My Agency Thoughts worksheet to help you identify any "I can" versus "I can't" thoughts you might have about actually engaging in those change efforts. You can use the same three steps to reflect on actual events that have caused you cultural stress in the past.

Culturally stressful event: Being followed in a store

You are shopping and get a feeling that the store clerks are following you around. Suddenly, the clerks approach you, and one says, "If you're not going to buy something, you need to leave. This isn't a hangout spot."

1. **What change efforts might you have the urge to make in this scenario?**

2. **Use the My Agency Thoughts worksheet on the next page to identify reasons you may or may not feel able to engage in these change efforts.**

3. **Based on your "I can" and "I can't" thinking above, would you feel able to engage in any change effort(s) in this situation?**

HOW TO KNOW WHEN YOU ARE EXPERIENCING AGENCY STRESS

In the preceding exercise, you were advised to check your BEAT reaction to an example of a culturally stressful event—specifically focusing in on the action urges and thoughts that were prompted by this example. Now you can delve a little deeper and bring your body sensations and emotions back into the picture, as these parts of your BEAT can help you notice how emotionally stressed you are by any lack of

My Agency Thoughts

EXPLANATIONS FOR AGENCY THINKING	WHAT TO THINK ABOUT	REASONS "I CAN"	REASONS "I CAN'T"
PERSONAL ABILITIES	Do you feel like you have the skills, traits, or abilities to engage in an effective change effort in this situation?		
ACCESS TO SUPPORT	Do you feel like you have any support from the people around you to engage in an effective change effort in this situation?		
COSTS VERSUS BENEFITS	Do you feel like the benefits of engaging in a change effort would outweigh the costs of not trying to do so in this situation?		

control or agency you might be feeling in a given moment. Here are the steps to follow for noticing agency stress.

1. **Describe a culturally stressful event that you've experienced.**

2. **Using your BEAT diagram, record your reactions to the culturally stressful event.**

3. **Assess the impact of the culturally stressful event on you.** Following are a few signs of agency stress to keep in mind when reviewing your BEAT reaction to see how you have been impacted by cultural stress.

   - **Figure out whether you've gotten stuck in an "I can't" mindset.** "I can't" thoughts are absolutely natural and make sense, especially if you've tried different things to influence your surroundings but feel discouraged by a lack of change. But sometimes a momentary "I can't" thought can turn into an "I can't" mindset. This is a sign that you generally feel like you don't have any power or control over a particular part of your life. When you notice yourself regularly having "I can't" thoughts in response to culturally stressful situations, consider exploring options for what you can still do in that situation to regain some sense of control and agency.

- **Notice whether you're starting to avoid stressful people or places.** It's natural to want to separate yourself from stressful people or places, especially when you feel powerless to change them. However, what happens when you feel that cultural stress is inescapable? What if you try to ignore a source of cultural stress but it keeps sneaking back into your mind? In such moments, you may feel unable to think of any options besides avoiding the source of cultural stress. When this happens, consider it a sign that you might benefit from exploring options for boosting your sense of agency and control.
- **Notice whether your change efforts have had unsatisfying results.** Let's say you come up with and actually engage in some change efforts, like educating someone about your experience or telling someone you will not be spoken to in a certain way. That's awesome, right? But what if these efforts do not get the results you hoped for? Say you tried to educate the person, but they responded in a dismissive or rude way. Making a change effort with an "I can" mindset is empowering, but it doesn't guarantee full satisfaction with the outcome. If you find yourself disappointed in the product of your efforts, step back and consider if it would be in your best interest to brainstorm new approaches to pursuing agency and control.

The preceding steps can increase your awareness of any agency stress you're experiencing by linking it to certain recognizable action urges and thoughts. Amia gained the following insights from using this worksheet.

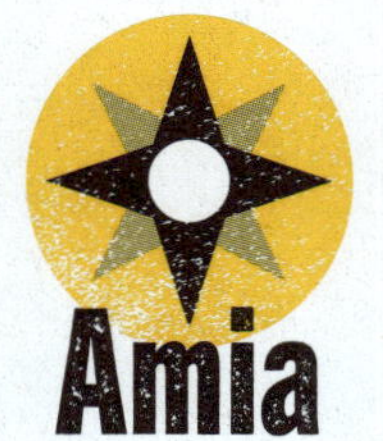

Amia's Effort to Practice Noticing Her Agency Stress

Amia was in her U.S. history class, and her teacher, Mr. Jones, was reviewing the modern U.S. wars. Mr. Jones began to discuss the events surrounding 9/11 and how they led to the "War on Terror." During class, a student named Rick asked a question about whether Muslims are still a threat to America. The teacher ignored the question and continued with the lecture. Amia felt this question was ridiculous and was surprised nothing more was said or done by the teacher or any classmate to educate Rick about the existence of peaceful and loving Muslim communities both in and outside of the U.S. After the class was dismissed, Rick approached Amia, an openly observant Muslim wearing hijab, and jokingly asked, "You aren't going to get upset one day and bomb our school, right?" Amia began tearing up, which prompted Rick to say, "C'mon, I'm just playing. Don't be so sensitive."

1. Describe the culturally stressful situation.

Where were you?	My history class
Who was present?	Classmates, teacher, and Rick
Describe the relationship or community stressor	Rick made insensitive comments about my faith, and no one stood up for me.

2. Using your BEAT diagram, record your reactions to the culturally stressful event.

- **Your urges:** any urges to engage in change efforts or avoidance when faced with this culturally stressful event
- **Your agency thoughts:** any "I can" or "I can't" thoughts you've been experiencing.
- **Your bodily sensations and emotions:** any body sensations or emotions you're experiencing in response to the culturally stressful event

Here is what Amia's BEAT diagram looked like.

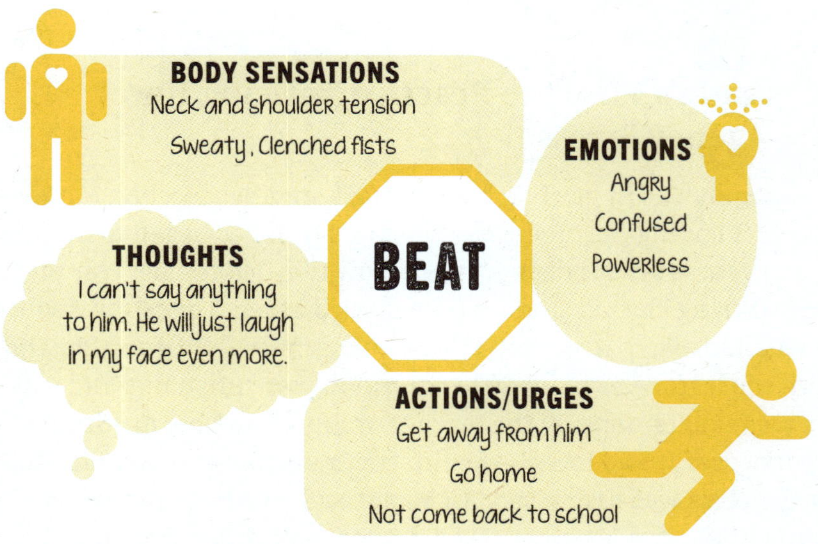

3. **Assess the impact of the culturally stressful event on you.** When looking at your BEAT diagram, do you notice yourself having any of the following?

Mostly "I can't" thoughts	● Yes	○ No
Avoidance urges/efforts	● Yes	○ No
Unsatisfactory change efforts	○ Yes	● No

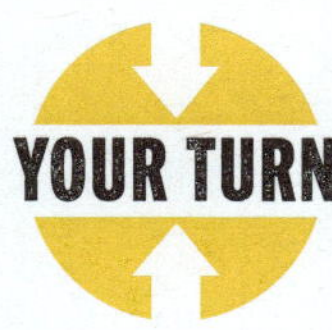

Use the same steps that Amia used to notice your agency stress any time you're wondering whether you're experiencing this type of cultural stress impact (see the worksheet on pages 130–131).

Power Up! Tips for Boosting Your Empowered Coping

Calling in your workbook navigators: If you answered "yes" to any of the signs of agency stress, you may find it helpful to talk to your workbook navigators about how you could boost your sense of agency or control in response to culturally stressful events. For example, you might ask them:

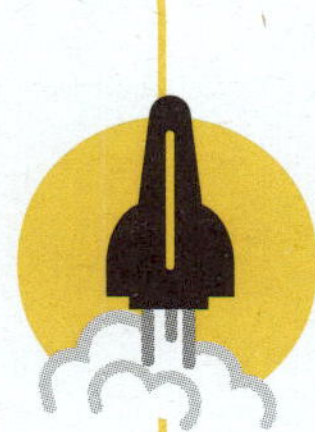

- What are some change efforts that you might make in this situation?
- What would help you have "I can" thoughts about engaging in a change effort?
- How would you boost your sense of control in this situation without resorting to avoiding or trying to ignore the sources of your stress?
- Are there ways to feel more in control of the situation even if your change efforts don't produce exactly the change you wanted?

Chapter 10: Recap and Reflect

RECAP

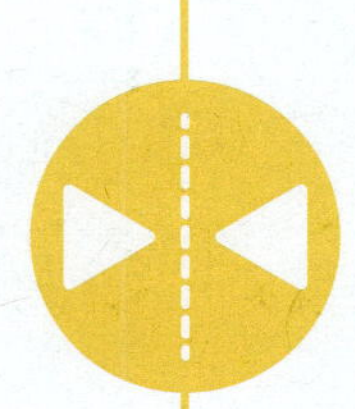

- In this chapter, you learned to use the **BEAT diagram** to help you observe when you are experiencing agency stress.
- Specifically, agency stress describes when your BEAT diagram includes mostly **"I can't" thoughts, strong avoidant urges/efforts,** or **feeling unsatisfied with the outcome** of your change efforts.

Noticing My Agency Stress

1. Describe the culturally stressful situation.

Where were you?	
Who was present?	
Describe the relationship or community stressor	

2. Using your BEAT diagram on the next page of this worksheet, record your reactions to the culturally stressful event.

- **Your urges:** any urges to engage in change efforts or avoidance when faced with this culturally stressful event
- **Your agency thoughts:** any "I can" or "I can't" thoughts you've been experiencing; use the My Agency Thoughts worksheet on page 126 if you need support with this
- **Your bodily sensations and emotions:** any body sensations or emotions you're experiencing in response to the culturally stressful event

3. Assess the impact of the culturally stressful event on you. When looking at your BEAT diagram, do you notice yourself having any of the following?

Mostly "I can't" thoughts	o Yes	o No
Avoidance urges/efforts	o Yes	o No
Unsatisfactory change efforts	o Yes	o No

(continued)

Noticing My Agency Stress *(page 2 of 2)*

BODY SENSATIONS

EMOTIONS

THOUGHTS

BEAT

ACTIONS/URGES

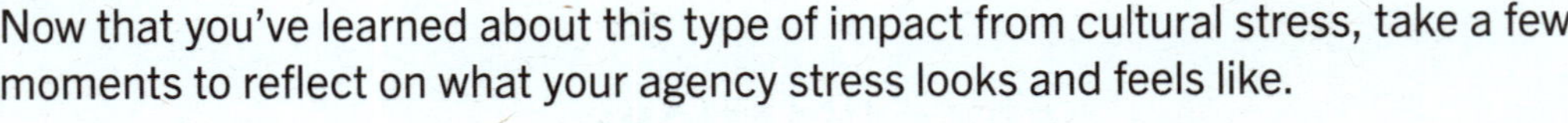

REFLECT

Now that you've learned about this type of impact from cultural stress, take a few moments to reflect on what your agency stress looks and feels like.

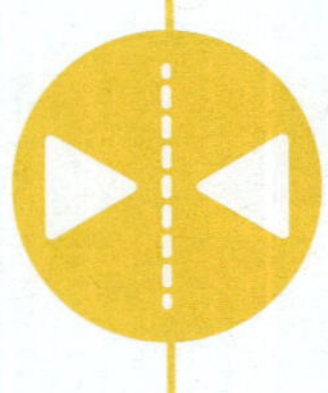

What types of culturally stressful events most often trigger agency stress for you?

Did you notice any particular body sensations or emotions that also occur when you're experiencing agency stress?

Do you ever criticize or judge yourself for your efforts to ignore or avoid the sources of stress or "I can't" thoughts in response to a culturally stressful event? If so, what does your self-criticism or self-judgment sound like?

11 How Can I Show Kindness and Understanding toward My Agency Stress?

When a POC sees or experiences an injustice, they can be flooded with thoughts critiquing how they responded to the situation. You know, asking yourself questions like:

- "Did I do the right thing?"
- "Did I represent my people well?"
- "Did I come off as weak?"

Importantly, how you answer these questions impacts not only the emotional stress you might feel over culturally stressful events but also the intensity of the agency stress. In Part Two, you were encouraged to practice self-compassion by learning to turn up the volume on your compassionate narrator. As you may remember, this narrator encourages you to show kindness and understanding toward the moment-to-moment experiences you have. Doing so helps you problem-solve how to cope with the realities of the moment you're experiencing.

In this chapter, you'll continue learning to use your compassionate narrator to catch any self-judgments that unfairly criticize your decision to (or not to) engage in change efforts when faced with cultural stress. You'll also learn to manage the stress caused by these judgments by showing yourself kindness while building understanding toward the true challenges that interfere with your sense of control and agency.

HOW TO SHOW YOURSELF KINDNESS AND UNDERSTANDING WHEN EXPERIENCING AGENCY STRESS

For many people subjected to cultural stress, self-criticism is a well-worn path. Just like any habit, taking a closer look at the mental, emotional, and behavioral process involved makes it easier to change. Here are the steps you can follow to break free from the ways self-criticism may hinder your empowered coping.

1. **Catch your judgments.** When looking back at moments when you did or didn't choose to make a change effort in response to culturally stressful events, it is important to acknowledge if there are any negative or overly critical self-judgments toward how you responded to your surroundings. This is important because these self-judgments can cause "I can't" thoughts to grow, cause "I can" thoughts to vanish, and rob you of the motivation to continue making change efforts. The following table provides some examples of self-judgments to spark insight (a version for you to fill in appears later in the chapter).

TYPES OF SELF-JUDGMENT	DESCRIPTION	EXAMPLES
CRITICAL LABELING	Using critical labels to describe how you handled or responded to a culturally stressful event (*Hint:* You may be experiencing this self-judgment if you use "*I am*" thinking.)	Because of how I responded: "*I am* so weak." "*I am* a pushover." "*I am* too sensitive." "*I am* an angry person."
SELF-BLAME	Taking most (if not all) of the responsibility for why the culturally stressful event happened or any outcomes from the event (*Hint:* You may be experiencing this self-judgment if you are mainly questioning "*What's wrong with me?*" or "*What did I do wrong?*")	"Why did I let them do this to me?" "I need to just work harder and stop letting these silly things get in my way." "If I wasn't so sensitive, I would have handled myself better."
OVERSIMPLIFIED COPING	Overlooking or minimizing the ways cultural stress can be difficult to manage or cope with (*Hint:* You may be experiencing this self-judgment if you are using "*should*" thinking.)	"I *should* have just tried harder." "I *should* have said more." "Why did I just sit there? I *should* have stood up for myself."

2. **Reflect on your reality.** While such judgments may alert you to your dissatisfaction or discouragement over how you did (or did not) attempt to stand up to an injustice, they also can cause you to overlook important details about the situation and leave you walking away with overly negative and critical perspectives of yourself and your capabilities. And although you may not be able to make these judgments completely go away, you can manage them by learning to acknowledge

the realities that complicate your responses to culturally stressful events. In the handout below are several prompts to help you take a step back and acknowledge different situational and personal realities that can make it hard to engage in efforts that truly lead to change, correction, and improvement (a version for you to fill in appears later in the chapter, but you might want to bookmark the handout to refer back to the "What to think about" prompts).

3. Compassionately state your reality. Whenever you mentally replay how you handled a culturally stressful event, it can be tempting to focus only on the self-judgments (step 1) and ignore the complicating realities surrounding the event (step 2). Even when you gain new perspectives from the reflection prompts in step 2, it can be hard to keep these new thoughts and feelings in mind as you move forward. So, after completing steps 1 and 2, one way to make sense of all of this

Acknowledging My Reality

MY REALITY	WHAT TO THINK ABOUT
Acknowledge the relationship or community stressors	For *relationship stressors,* describe the details of your social interaction that caused you to feel judged or treated differently because of your racial and cultural background. For *community stressors,* describe the details of the community space that caused you to feel unfairly denied an opportunity or unsupported because of your racial and cultural background. Have you ever been in a situation like this before? How might any newness of these stressors influence how you acted or responded?
Acknowledge the emotional stress	How might the body sensations and emotions you felt in response to the culturally stressful event have impacted your ability to act or respond in the way that you wanted?
Acknowledge the coping challenges	Are there any details of the culturally stressful event that impacted or hindered your ability to act in the way you might have wanted? How might other people similarly struggle to take action if faced with the same culturally stressful event?
Acknowledge my change efforts	Though it may be tempting to focus on what you didn't do, list any ways you still tried to influence change when dealing with culturally stressful events. If unable to think of any change efforts you did make, how might the realities stated above, such as your emotional stress or the coping challenges, have made it difficult to engage in a change effort?
Acknowledge others' responsibility	What ways do the people around you and the community spaces around you need to change, be corrected, or be improved? What responsibility do others have for limiting your exposure to culturally stressful events moving forward?
Acknowledge my learning	If you ever face a similar culturally stressful event again in the future, what did you learn from this experience that might help you act or respond in a way that you might feel prouder of in the future?

information in a way that will stick with you is to lovingly summarize to yourself *what you hoped for in that situation, what made your hopes difficult to achieve in that situation,* and *where you want to go from here.*

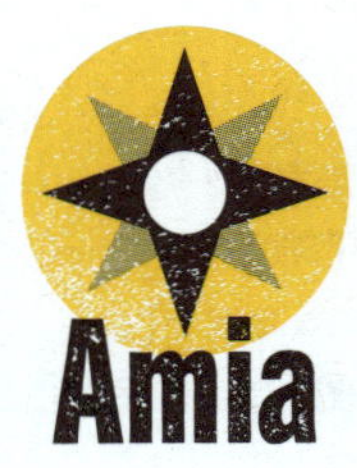

Amia's Efforts to Show Kindness and Understanding toward Her Agency Stress

When Amia's classmate rudely expressed negative judgments about her Muslim faith in a history class and then criticized her tearful response, her first instinct was to escape their conversation. And that's just what she did: She remained silent and then walked away in tears. Afterward, Amia struggled with her silence and judged herself for not telling Rick to stop disrespecting her faith in this way or even educating him about the offensive nature of his words.

1. **Catch your judgments.** Amia noticed the following self-judgments.

TYPES OF SELF-JUDGMENT	DESCRIBE YOUR SELF-JUDGMENTS
CRITICAL LABELING	I am such a pushover for not saying anything.
SELF-BLAME	Rick talks to me that way because I am an easy target. It's because I never speak up for myself.
OVERSIMPLIFIED COPING	I shouldn't have just walked away like a punk. I should have just told him off.

2. **Reflect on your reality.** By reflecting on the prompts, Amia started to notice her focus shift away from dwelling on the overly critical self-judgements from step 1. She began to notice her compassionate narrator getting louder. Remember, Amia's efforts to think about her reality do not erase her frustrations about how she responded or instantly grant her more control over her culturally stressful surroundings. Instead, she is learning to consider how and why she responded in the ways she did. All of this is very important because it can help her create more realistic coping plans for finding her sense of control and agency at school.

Acknowledge the relationship or community stressors:
The relationship stressor is feeling like my faith was discussed unfairly in that class and feeling unsure why Rick felt the need to target me. And I guess the community stressor is feeling my school is so unsupportive—like nobody said anything about Rick's nonsense. I've heard of people being this ignorant. But I have never experienced something like this before.

Acknowledge the emotional stress:

I was so shocked when he said what he said. I felt so surprised and caught off guard. I kind of froze and just didn't know what to say.

Acknowledge the coping challenges:

I felt hindered by being in a class full of people with everyone staring at me. It felt like so much pressure—like people were just waiting to see how the little Brown girl would respond. And then being caught off guard again after class when I was still upset about what had happened. All of that just made it so hard to think clearly and decide what to do.

Acknowledge your change efforts:

I guess it makes sense that I couldn't find the right words to say to Rick. I guess I felt I needed to get away from him while I was feeling so overwhelmed.

Acknowledge others' responsibility:

I think my teacher should have noticed that Rick's comment was inappropriate. He should have said something. Also, Rick needs to do better. He needs to check himself and know that everything in your head doesn't need to be said.

Acknowledge your learning:

I learned that I don't like my faith being talked about like this. I learned that I can struggle to speak up in moments like this. Not sure exactly what I could have done differently though. I guess walking away allowed me to get away from Rick so I could make sense of what happened. But I still don't like that I haven't said anything to him or anyone about what happened.

3. Compassionately state your reality. Here is how Amia tried to state her reality in a way that can help keep the volume of her compassionate narrator turned up as she figures out how she wants to respond to her interactions with Rick.

In this situation, I had hoped I would (or they would):

I hoped I would speak up and defend myself in the class and when talking to Rick. I had hoped my teacher and classmates would support me more.

In this situation, it was difficult to achieve my hopes and wishes because:

In this situation, it was difficult to achieve my hopes and wishes because: Speaking up in moments like this is hard for me. Plus, I have never been in a situation like this before. And it's hard to know exactly what to say when you feel so much pressure.

Moving forward, if I face a similar culturally stressful event, I hope I will:

Moving forward, if I face a similar culturally stressful event, I guess I hope I will say something to my teacher. But I guess that depends on the teacher. I don't exactly know. I just hope I will speak up somehow.

Moving forward, I hope to become more confident in my ability to:

Moving forward, I hope to become more confident in my ability to: Speak up to people. Or at least let someone know that I didn't like how I was treated.

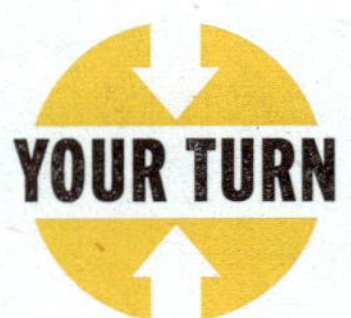

The three steps you've just read about offer you several alternatives to self-criticism when experiencing agency stress. As you can imagine, this coping skill is not always easy or may not immediately feel very comforting. Sometimes taking a step back and acknowledging the realities that seem beyond your control can trigger more anger, frustrations, anxiety, or sadness. But, as the saying goes, "We got to keep it all the way real." When you don't honor the complicating reality that impacts your reactions to cultural stress, you're left with putting all the blame and responsibility on your own shoulders while ignoring the ways cultural stress continues to frustrate even the best and brightest efforts.

Use the prompts below to help you turn up your compassionate narrator any time you face agency stress—especially in moments when you feel critical of your change efforts.

1. **Catch your judgments.** Describe any critical self-judgments you have toward how you handle a culturally stressful event in the worksheet on the facing page.

2. **Reflect on your reality.** Fill in the worksheet on page 140. Use the "What to think about" ideas in the handout on page 135.

Power Up! Tips for Boosting Your Empowered Coping
Here are some ideas to help if you find completing step 2 difficult.

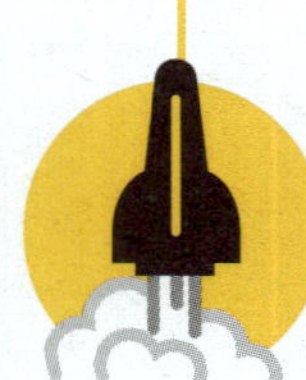

- **Cope with emotional stress.** Consider using a soothing effort from Chapter 8 as your first compassionate response if you notice any emotional stress while trying to use these steps.
- **Start small.** Pick one or two reflection prompts from step 2 that feel most appropriate for the situation you are in.
- **Revisit these prompts.** You may have to return to these reflection prompts multiple times before you notice yourself developing more kindness and understanding toward your experience.
- **Journal and seek support.** You may even find it helpful to use these reflection prompts to journal in a notebook or to explore these prompts with any of your workbook navigators to see what kinds of responses they come up with.

3. **Compassionately state your reality.** Now state your reality (page 141), acknowledging the hardships that influenced your responses to culturally stressful events.

My Critical Self-Judgments toward How I Handled a Culturally Stressful Event

TYPES OF SELF-JUDGMENT	DESCRIPTION	DESCRIBE YOUR SELF-JUDGMENTS
CRITICAL LABELING	Using critical labels to describe how you handled or responded to a culturally stressful event (*Hint:* You may be experiencing this self-judgment if you use "*I am*" thinking.)	
SELF-BLAME	Taking most (if not all) of the responsibility for why the culturally stressful event happened or any outcomes from the event (*Hint:* You may be experiencing this self-judgment if you are mainly questioning "*What's wrong with me?*" or "*What did I do wrong?*")	
OVERSIMPLIFIED COPING	Overlooking or minimizing the ways cultural stress can be difficult to manage or cope with (*Hint:* You may be experiencing this self-judgment if you are using "*should*" thinking.)	
OTHER?		

What's My Reality?

Acknowledge the relationship or community stressor:

Acknowledge the emotional stress:

Acknowledge the coping challenges:

Acknowledge your change efforts:

Acknowledge others' responsibility:

Acknowledge your learning:

Self-Compassion toward My Reality

In this situation, I had hoped I would (or they would):

In this situation, it was difficult to achieve my hopes and wishes because:

Moving forward, if I face a similar culturally stressful event, I hope I will:

Moving forward, I hope to become more confident in my ability to:

Chapter 11: Recap and Reflect

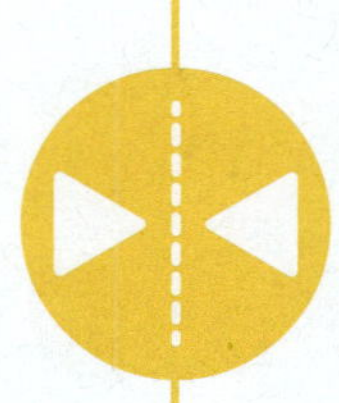

RECAP

- In Chapter 5, you learned that **self-compassion** describes efforts to show kindness and understanding toward the body sensations, emotions, action urges, and thoughts (BEAT) experienced in any given moment.
- Also, you learned that developing and growing your self-compassionate narrator will help you cope with and heal from culturally stressful situations.

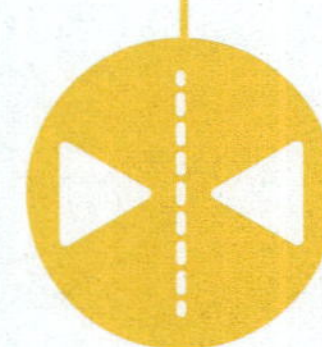

- Some ways to practice self-compassion for agency stress are to:
  - Notice any critical judgments toward your responses to the culturally stressful event(s).
  - Reflect on the realities that complicated your responses to the culturally stressful event(s).
  - Compassionately state the truth surrounding your responses to the culturally stressful event(s)—*what you hoped for, what made your hopes difficult to achieve,* and *where you want to go from here.*

REFLECT

Before moving forward, let's take a moment to think about what you learned about self-compassion and how you hope this skill can help you cope with agency stress. To do so, answer the questions below.

What does **self-compassion** mean to you, and how can it be helpful when you are experiencing agency stress?

In addition to what you learned in this chapter, are there other ways that you have learned to show kindness and understanding toward your behavioral responses to culturally stressful events?

How can practicing **self-compassion** enhance your ability to cope with any agency stress you experience moving forward?

12 My Agency Stress Coping Assessment

Many conversations about coping with cultural stress focus on handling the emotional impact (as in Part Two of this workbook). But true empowerment is more than riding the wave of emotional pain. It has to include gaining some sense of *agency* and *control* over your experiences while in the relationships and community spaces that are the source of your stress.

This book takes a balanced approach to this discussion. Think of it as a balancing act that requires you to prioritize change and resilience:

- As we've been discussing, **change efforts** include clarifying what you want to address about the relationship or community space and creating an action plan to change, correct, or improve your surroundings. Remember to think of change through the lens of your *efforts,* not solely *outcomes.* Why? You have the greatest control over the effort you choose to (or not to) engage in. That's what Part Three is all about—clarifying what efforts remain within your control. And, by focusing only on the outcomes of fighting for change, you can lose sight of what empowered efforts you have made (and can still make) in the face of injustice.

- You also need tools to help you maintain a meaningful presence within spaces that are slow to change. This is where your **resilience efforts** come into the picture. While you await the change you want to see, you also need useful and meaningful resilience efforts that remain within your control. These efforts help you take steps toward achieving meaningful goals within social spaces despite the culturally stressful events that keep appearing, like potholes in the road forward.

AGENCY EFFORTS	MOTIVATIONS	EXAMPLES
CHANGE EFFORTS	• Try to change or correct people or places responsible for cultural stress • Improve the experience of POCs within culturally stressful surroundings	• Confront and communicate • Seek advocacy • Organize/join social actions
RESILIENCE EFFORTS	• Endure cultural stress caused by people or places • Sustain effort and progress toward your goals despite cultural stress	• Clarify personal goals • Make efforts toward goals • Find support for your goals

In this chapter you will assess whether you currently feel able to engage in any of the agency efforts described above that feel meaningful and effective when faced with cultural stress. If not, you'll be able to turn to the chapters recommended at the end of this chapter that may help you improve your empowered coping with agency stress. Please thoughtfully and carefully complete the next few exercises to help you understand these important insights.

HOW TO USE THE AGENCY STRESS COPING DIAGRAM

To help you strengthen your coping skills for experiences of agency stress, the next two chapters will help you practice each skill displayed in the **agency stress coping diagram.** In Chapter 13, you'll have the opportunity to explore your options for changing, correcting, or improving your culturally stressful surroundings. In Chapter 14, you can explore options for maintaining a meaningful presence while remaining in relationships and community spaces that are culturally stressful.

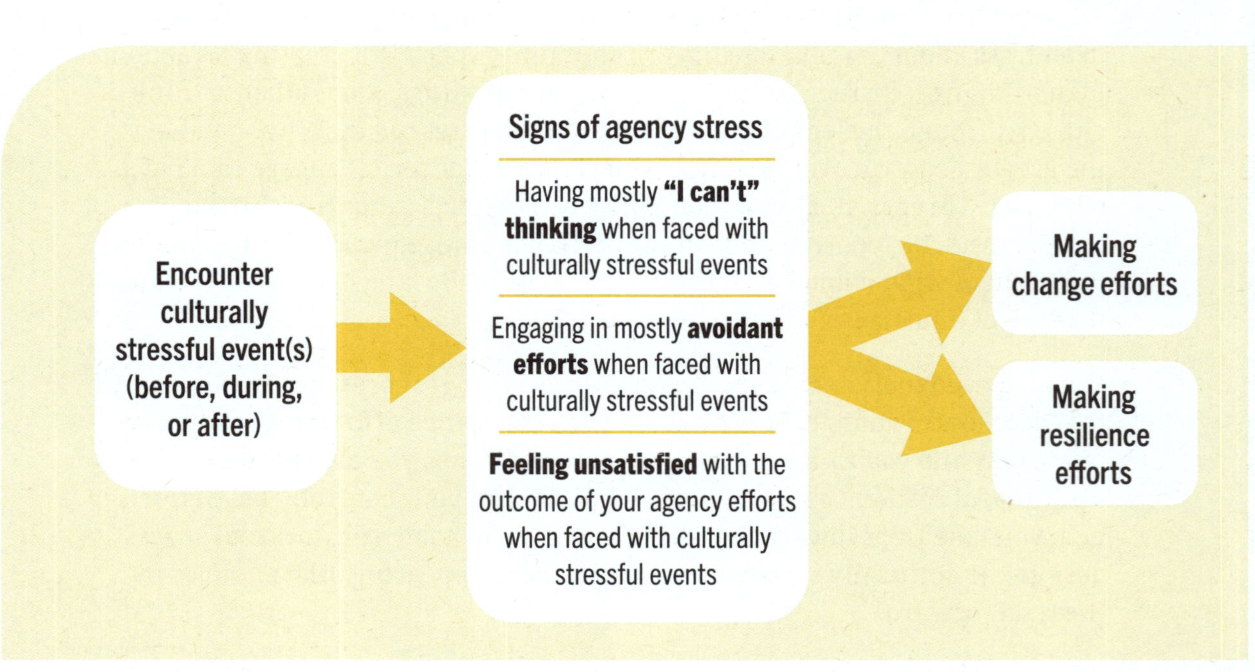

Here are the steps to take to discover whether you've used any of the coping skills in the diagram on page 144 when faced with a culturally stressful event.

1. **Identify a culturally stressful event.** Describe a past, present, or anticipated culturally stressful event that caused you to experience agency stress. If you have any difficulty thinking of an example, look back at your My Relationship and Community Map (page 33).

2. **Reflect on the agency stress coping diagram.** Review the prompts below for a quick preview of each coping decision and see if you can think of any examples of how you've already practiced each type of coping.

CHANGE EFFORTS	Did you try to change, correct, or improve your social or community spaces to reduce your exposure to cultural stresses within these spaces?	○ Yes ○ No ○ Not sure
RESILIENCE EFFORTS	Did you make any intentional decisions to continue pursuing important goals while remaining within culturally stressful surroundings?	○ Yes ○ No ○ Not sure
Are there any additional ways that you try to cope with agency stress?		

3. **Reflect on the result of your efforts.** Let's get your thoughts on how you felt you handled the agency stress from this culturally stressful event.

Were you pleased with how you handled any agency stress you experienced?	○ Yes ○ No ○ Somewhat
Why or why not?	

Chapter 12: Recap and Reflect

RECAP

- When you notice agency stress, you can search for ways to regain your sense of control and power by **balancing your change and resilience efforts** within that particular setting.

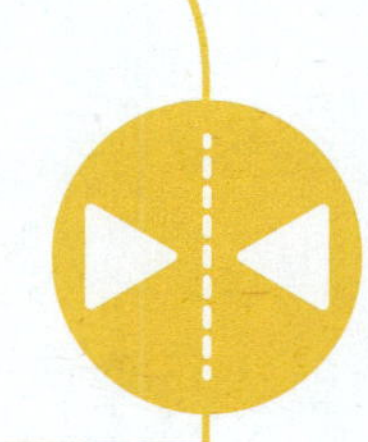

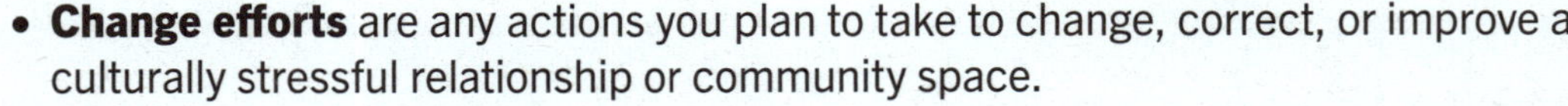

- **Change efforts** are any actions you plan to take to change, correct, or improve a culturally stressful relationship or community space.

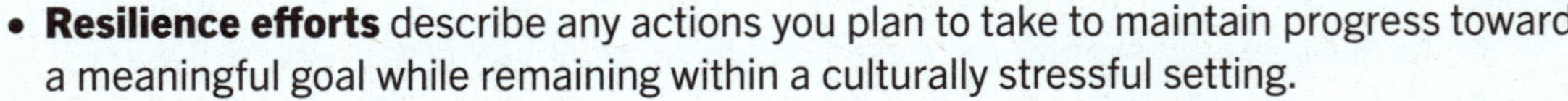

- **Resilience efforts** describe any actions you plan to take to maintain progress toward a meaningful goal while remaining within a culturally stressful setting.

REFLECT

Use the questionnaire below to help you determine which of the remaining chapters in Part Three you are most interested in reviewing.

IMPACT FROM AGENCY STRESS	RESPONSES	CHAPTER IN PART THREE
Are you ever unsure when or how to make efforts to change, correct, or improve your culturally stressful surroundings?	○ Yes ○ No	**If "yes," go to Chapter 13 (on how to make change efforts)**
Are you ever unsure how to continue progressing toward meaningful goals when having to remain within social or community spaces when change, correction, or improvement is difficult?	○ Yes ○ No	**If "yes," go to Chapter 14 (on how to make resilience efforts)**

13 How Can I Change or Improve Stressful Surroundings?

As you worked your way through the first three chapters of Part Three, you may have realized that you have certain instincts about how to address agency stress. Maybe your natural instinct in the face of culturally stressful events is to put your head down and focus on doing what you can to achieve important goals (making resilience efforts). Or your gut tells you to ignore the existence of cultural stress around you (making avoidant efforts). In these cases, you might find engaging in change efforts quite challenging. In contrast, if your reflexive choice is to resist the status quo or to be the squeaky wheel that challenges the powers that be to do better and be better for POCs, you're probably more comfortable with change efforts than the other coping efforts.

In either case, when you do choose to go for change, correction, or improvement, you're encouraged to make that decision thoughtfully and carefully. Such decision making invites you to take into account when it makes sense to push for change and when it makes sense to take a break to conserve your energy, so you can focus on other goals within your culturally stressful surroundings. That's what this chapter is designed to help you with. It breaks the process of pursuing change into smaller steps that help you:

- Brainstorm ideas for pursuing the change you want to see
- Determine when making change efforts is the most empowered coping decision for you

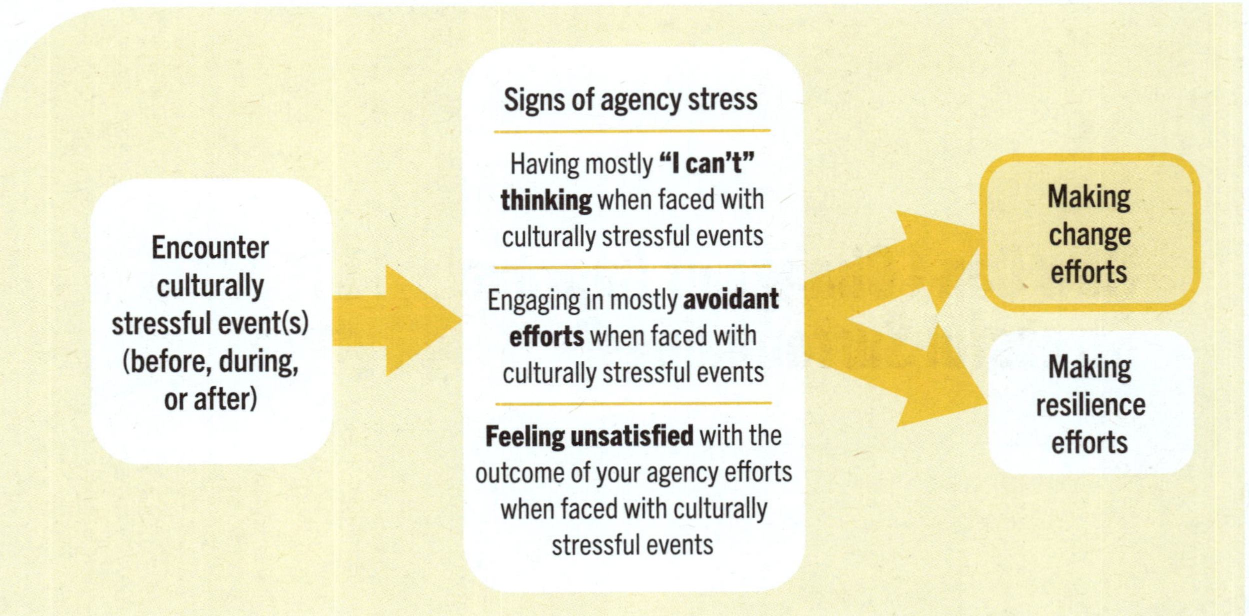

HOW TO PURSUE CHANGE IN YOUR RELATIONSHIPS AND COMMUNITY SPACES

This chapter will help you create a plan for engaging in **change efforts** by identifying your change goals, brainstorming efforts for pursuing those goals, weighing the pros and cons of specific change efforts, carefully evaluating your options, and finally coming up with a plan for making change efforts. Here are the steps in a little more detail.

1. **Identify your change goals.** The first step is to ask yourself, "What do I want to change, correct, or improve about my culturally stressful surroundings?" Your answer might focus on changes you want to see in a relationship where you feel unfairly judged or mistreated because of your racial and cultural background (relationship stressor). Such relationships can be with family members, friends, authority figures, or even a stranger. You can also think of change goals that are directed toward parts of your community that do not offer fair access to opportunities or the support you need to achieve your goals (community stressor). Such goals could apply to policies within a school or workspace, certain resources that you feel should be made more accessible, or even laws that you wish were changed.

2. **Brainstorm change efforts.** Reaching a goal isn't like taking one huge leap from intention and landing right at the desired outcome. It's important to figure out what steps you need to take to get to the change you want. This chapter offers

three ways to pursue your change goals—confront and communicate, seek support and advocacy, and engage in activism. You'll find tip sheets to help you brainstorm about taking these routes on pages 150–154.

3. Consider the costs of fighting for change. Choosing to invest time and energy into change efforts rarely comes with no costs or unwanted consequences. To make empowered decisions about which change goals to pursue, you have to anticipate the potential costs and whether you're willing to take them on. What if confronting a friend could cause you to lose the friendship? Are you still willing to commit to that change effort? What if the fight for change goes on for days, weeks, or even years? Investing a lot of time into social justice and activism efforts could leave you emotionally worn down, exhausted, and possibly disheartened. Would you be able to continue the fight? Will you need extra support to help you manage any costs from your actions? You'll want to consider these four types of costs you may encounter when pursuing change:

- **Social costs**—feeling that engaging in any of the change efforts you brainstormed will be met with rejection, criticism, or negative judgment
- **Resource costs**—feeling that engaging in any of the change efforts you brainstormed will lead to a removal or denial of needed or wanted resources
- **Safety costs**—feeling that engaging in any of the change efforts you brainstormed will be met with threatened or experienced physical harm
- **Emotional costs**—feeling that engaging any of the change efforts you brainstormed may cause you overwhelming bodily and emotional discomfort

4. Evaluate your options. This is usually the hardest step in planning for change. You have to answer the question "Do the possible benefits of my actions outweigh the possible unwanted outcomes?" This is an extremely personal question that can elicit many different answers. To help you evaluate your options, I encourage you to compare the pros and cons of potentially engaging in at least two change efforts.

5. Decide whether to make a change effort. Your evaluation of the pros and cons can enable you to decide whether putting your change effort into action is worth any costs you've considered. Step 5 is where you decide to either:

- **Engage** in change efforts—choose to make a change effort while coping ahead for any anticipated costs you listed in step 3
- **Not engage** in change efforts—choose to engage in a resilience effort instead (see Chapter 14)

TIP SHEETS FOR MAKING CHANGE EFFORTS

Tip Sheet: Confront and Communicate

Even when you may desperately want to confront or educate others about their culturally stressful behavior, you may feel like you just don't know what to say. This tip sheet offers a few statements or questions that are intended to help you brainstorm options for confronting and communicating with culturally stressful people around you. The table below is divided into two categories—communicating boundaries and educating others. Take a look and see if any of these options might help you think of ways to confront people who are treating you insensitively.

COMMUNICATING BOUNDARIES		EDUCATING OTHERS	
Encouraging others to treat you fairly and respectfully		**Sharing information about yourself or your background**	
"I don't like when you do that. Please don't do or say that again."	"How would you respond if someone cut in front of you?"	"I gotta keep it real. What you just did makes me feel very uncomfortable."	"Do you think that all [describe your background] are supposed to like the same things?"
"Excuse you! I am standing here."	"I am curious. Would you remain in a conversation where someone speaks to you like you just spoke to me?"	"When I heard you say or do ________, that doesn't apply to me."	"What makes you think someone like me can't care about that?"
"I will not remain in this conversation if you continue to speak to me in this way."	"Would you keep showing up if you didn't feel supported, heard, or valued?"	"I actually care a lot about [describe your interests or values]."	"Have you spent much time getting to know [describe your background] people?"
"My time is precious. I will not continue to invest my time and effort if I do not receive more support."	List any other statements/questions that can be used to **communicate boundaries:**	"What you said doesn't describe all [describe your background]."	List any other statements/questions that can be used to **educate others:**

COMMUNICATING BOUNDARIES		EDUCATING OTHERS	
"Do you speak to everyone that way or just someone who looks like me?"	List any other statements/questions that can be used to **communicate boundaries:**	"How would you respond if someone did what you just did to me?	List any other statements/questions that can be used to **educate others:**

Power Up! Tips for Boosting Your Empowered Coping

- Consider reviewing these options with your workbook navigators to see if there are any additional statements/questions they have used.
- Knowing what you could say and feeling confident you can say it are not the same thing. Think about the following to increase your confidence in advance.
  - What would it look or sound like if you were to communicate your boundaries or educate others *confidently?*
  - What tone of voice and body language would give you the *best chance to be heard and clearly understood?*
  - What can you do to *maintain your self-respect* as you communicate—especially if the other person does not have a satisfactory response?
  - Consider asking your workbook navigators to role-play a culturally stressful interaction and practice using one of these statements/questions, so that you can think through your delivery and cope ahead for any responses you may receive.

Tip Sheet: Seek Support and Advocacy

When dealing with cultural stress, social supports can help you explore your BEAT reactions, feel affirmed in your empowered responses, and problem-solve your next steps. One additional resource your social supports can offer is advocacy. Sometimes you may benefit from having others to lean on while you pursue your change goals. To identify potential supporters, it can be helpful to know what you're looking for. Use this Tip Sheet to help you identify the people around you who you may be willing to ask to support you in your fight for change.

1. **What are you looking for in an advocate?** *Circle or check off* the qualities you feel are necessary for you to feel comfortable seeking support.

- ☐ **Understands me:** I feel heard and as if my experience matters
- ☐ **Nonjudgmental:** Someone who offers support without judging my responses as good or bad
- ☐ **Trustworthy:** I have confidence that what I share will be kept private
- ☐ **Similar experiences:** Someone who has a background and experiences similar to mine
- ☐ **Supportive:** Someone who offers me consistent support
- ☐ **Good listener:** Someone who listens with limited distraction and shows interest in what I am saying
- ☐ **Validating:** Someone who maintains space for and tries to understand my emotions
- ☐ **Values aligned:** Someone who cares about similar things
- ☐ **Respectful:** Someone who respects the things I care about (especially the differences between our values)
- ☐ **Problem solver:** Someone who is helpful in generating solutions for problems
- ☐ **Empathy:** Someone who demonstrates understanding toward my emotions and experience
- ☐ **Genuine:** Someone who is authentic and "keeps it real" with me
- ☐ **Open-minded:** Someone who is able to see multiple perspectives without being quick to pass judgment
- ☐ **Showing up:** Someone who is available when called on
- ☐ **Makes me feel safe:** I feel able to be my authentic self around this person
- ☐ **Knowledgeable ("woke"):** Someone who knows cultural stress exists and just gets it
- ☐ **Good advocate:** Someone who is willing to use their power or authority to support me
- ☐ Other: ____________________
- ☐ Other: ____________________

2. Identify potential advocates. In Chapter 2 you were asked to create a My Relationship and Community Map. Take a look back at the relationships you listed throughout your map (page 33). In the table below, write down one or two people who seem to represent any of the qualities you circled or checked off above.

POTENTIAL ADVOCATE'S NAME	THEIR ADVOCATE QUALITIES

Tip Sheet: Engaging in Activism

Sometimes you may not feel able to directly change the dynamics in a particular relationship to make it less culturally stressful. Or maybe you doubt that correcting someone's misperceptions will be truly impactful. Another change effort focuses on improving your community more broadly by investing time and energy into social actions that feel meaningful. The upcoming table lists a variety of activism initiatives you might want to participate in. Take a look and see if any initiatives seem interesting.

As you review the options in the table, keep in mind what goals you hope to achieve by engaging in activism. Ask yourself, "What ways am I most interested in making efforts to improve or give back to my community?" Then take a quick glance back at the strengths section of your Who Am I? diagram from Chapter 1 (page 14) to help you consider which activism initiatives best align with your abilities.

1. **Identify your change goal.** In what ways are you most interested in making efforts to improve or give back to your community?

2. **Identify your abilities.** What abilities do you want to use to support your efforts to achieve your change goals?

3. **Choose your social action.** Choose a social action that you think best utilizes the abilities you just selected and that may help you make an effort toward your change goal.

Fundraising	**Social justice activism**	**Create a community project**	**Socially conscious artistic expression**
Raise and donate money to organizations that support social issues you care about	*Organize/join protests or marches about social issues that you care about*	*Start a service group or club to address a social issue within your community*	*Create and showcase art about your story or that raises awareness about social issues*
Community education	**Youth councils**	**Letter writing**	**Create an awareness campaign**
Organize educational opportunities, like workshops or panel discussions, for your community to learn new information about a social issue	*Join/participate in organizations or community meetings that allow your voice to be heard*	*Draft letters to authority figures, such as your elected officials, to raise awareness or request policy changes*	*Create social media, blogs, or photography about social issues*

Mentoring

Find opportunities to mentor and support younger generations within your community

Political engagement

Register to vote, support campaigns for politicians who support social issues you care about

Volunteer

Tutor, run food drives, or volunteer at a nonprofit organization

Affinity groups

Create, organize, or participate in support groups that focus on social issues related to your racial and cultural background

Media activism

Use social media to post information about social issues and join broader social movements with reposts and hashtags

Create your own:

Community cleanup

Clean up or organize community activities in hopes of improving community spaces that are important to you

Create your own:

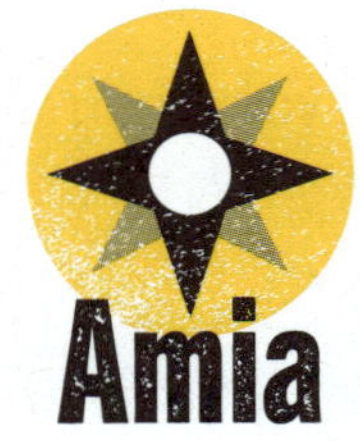

Amia's Plan for Making Change Efforts

Remember Amia's interactions with Rick in their history class? (If not, look back at Chapter 10.) Amia's natural reaction to Rick's offensive comments was to avoid and escape the classroom and Rick. However, as you saw in Chapter 11, she hopes to find change efforts to help her manage any future culturally stressful events. Here is how Amia used the exercises in this chapter to help create a plan for achieving this goal.

1. **Identify your change goals.** Check out Amia's change goals.

CHANGE GOALS TO CONSIDER	RESPONSES	MY CHANGE GOALS AND REASONS
Change relationship(s) *Are there any issues you want to address, boundaries you want to set, or information you want to share to change or improve a culturally stressful relationship?*	● Yes ○ No ○ Unsure	I really wish I could tell my teacher to speak up and correct any ignorant comments that are made about my culture. I also want to show Rick and all of my classmates that Muslim people are kind, friendly, and peaceful.
Change community space(s) *Are there ways you want to contribute to the improvement of your community that may reduce your (or others) exposure to culturally stressful events?*	● Yes ○ No ○ Unsure	It would be cool to help my school find ways to celebrate my Muslim culture.
Any other change goals that you have?	○ Yes ● No ○ Unsure	

2. Brainstorm change efforts. Here are Amia's ideas for change efforts in each category.

1. I could pursue my change goal by . . . using the confront and communicate strategy to talk with my teacher about what happened in class or talk to Rick about how disrespectful his comments were.
2. I could pursue my change goal by . . . seeking support and advocacy from my history teacher by asking that he be more mindful of any misinformation shared about my religion during class discussions.
3. I could pursue my change goal by . . . speaking with one of my school counselors about any school programming that can be created to support Muslim students. Maybe an afterschool club or something like that.

3. Consider the cost of fighting for change. From Amia's responses below, you can see that her interests in pursuing change do not come without concern of running into unwanted consequences.

Describe any **social costs** you are concerned about experiencing:	I am worried that if I stand up to Rick he might get really upset, argue away all my points, or possibly spread rumors about how much of a crybaby I am.
Describe any **resource costs** you are concerned about experiencing:	A girl at my mosque told me that a professor at her college did not like being called out by a student. She told me that this professor started grading the student more harshly and was less willing to help them. I guess I am worried about my history teacher doing that to me.
Describe any **safety costs** you are concerned about experiencing:	I am not really that concerned about being physically harmed. But I know this is a possibility. I have heard stories about people being physically harmed for standing up for their faith.
Describe any **emotional costs** you are concerned about experiencing:	It's already hard enough for me to go to school here. So standing up for myself kind of feels like I am just going to make school even more stressful and uncomfortable for me.

4. Evaluate your options. Amia used the worksheet on the next page to help her weigh the costs and benefits of pursuing two of the change efforts she brainstormed.

POSSIBLE CHANGE EFFORTS	WHAT IS *MOST HELPFUL* ABOUT THIS OPTION?	WHAT IS *LEAST HELPFUL* ABOUT THIS OPTION?
1. Talking to my history teacher	-He might support me more in class. -He will understand how students like me feel during these class discussions. -He might change his teaching style.	-He may get annoyed and upset with me for saying something. -He may grade me harshly. -He may not write me a letter of recommendation for college.
2. Speaking with school counselor about supportive programming	-I may find more people who are friendly. -Maybe there are other students who would benefit from such programming. -I might feel more comfortable at my school.	-My counselor might say no. -There may not be other students who are interested.

5. Decide whether to make a change effort. After carefully thinking through the pros and cons in step 4, Amia decided to first talk with her school counselor about creating a more affirming and supportive space for Muslim students—or at least creating a space where interested students can politely and supportively discuss cultural similarities and differences. For her, doing so would still represent a change effort that prioritizes her goal of improving her school environment. Importantly, this decision also considers Amia's concerns of retaliation that could result from confronting and communicating with her history teacher or her classmate Rick.

DESCRIBE YOUR EFFORT	WHEN DO YOU WANT TO PRACTICE?	COPE AHEAD PLAN
CHANGE EFFORT 1: Research ways other schools have supported Muslim students	I can begin looking things up on my phone today and then maybe find some time over the weekend to do a more complete search.	I already have a lot of school stuff on my plate, so it may be stressful to add another task like this to my plate. I will try to set a time limit on how long I research so I make sure I can focus on other things.
CHANGE EFFORT 2: Talk with school counselor about ideas	I'll stop by her office tomorrow to find a time when we can meet about this.	I guess I should prepare myself for the emotional hit if she says no. Or if she discourages me from doing this. Maybe I can use Chapter 8 of this workbook to help me think of ways to soothe my emotions if this happens.

DESCRIBE YOUR EFFORT	WHEN DO YOU WANT TO PRACTICE?	COPE AHEAD PLAN
CHANGE EFFORT 3: Ask school counselor for support	I'll ask for her support whenever we get to meet about this.	Again, I'll prepare myself emotionally if she seems unsupportive and possibly ask if she knows of another school staff member who could help me.

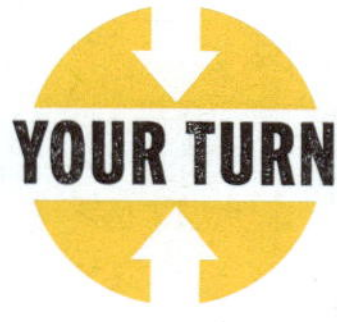

First, describe a culturally stressful event that you want to focus on for the remainder of this chapter. This can be a past, present, or anticipated event. Then follow the steps to help you think through what change efforts could look like in response to the culturally stressful event you describe.

1. Identify your change goals. In an ideal world, what do you wish you could change, correct, or improve about your culturally stressful surroundings?

My Change Goals

CHANGE GOALS TO CONSIDER	RESPONSES	MY CHANGE GOALS AND REASONS
Change relationship(s) *Are there any issues you want to address, boundaries you want to set, or information you want to share to change or improve a culturally stressful relationship?*	○ Yes ○ No ○ Unsure	
Change community space(s) *Are there ways you want to contribute to the improvement of your community that may reduce your (or others) exposure to culturally stressful events?*	○ Yes ○ No ○ Unsure	
Do you have any other change goals? *If yes, add them at right.*	○ Yes ○ No ○ Unsure	

2. **Brainstorm change efforts.** Anytime you have a goal you want to pursue, it's important to brainstorm steps toward achieving this goal. Pick at least one change goal from step 1 and think of at least three change efforts you could make toward pursuing your goal. If you have difficulty thinking of any change efforts, look back at the Tip Sheets beginning on page 150.

My Possible Change Efforts

1. I could pursue my change goal by. . . .

2. I could pursue my change goal by. . . .

3. I could pursue my change goal by. . . .

3. **Consider the costs of fighting for change.** Below, describe any costs you anticipate incurring from engaging in any of the *change efforts* you just brainstormed.

What Are the Costs of Fighting for Change?

Describe any **social costs** you are concerned about experiencing:	
Describe any **resource costs** you are concerned about experiencing:	
Describe any **safety costs** you are concerned about experiencing:	
Describe any **emotional costs** you are concerned about experiencing:	
Describe any other costs you are concerned about experiencing:	

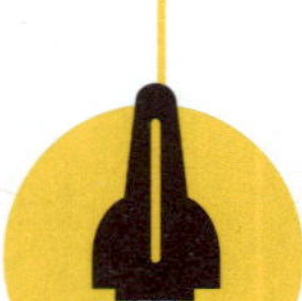

Power Up! Tips for Boosting Your Empowered Coping

Have you ever heard the term *privilege?* Those viewed as "privileged" have access to certain resources, rights, and advantages that others do not have. There are times when our change efforts are focused on changing, correcting, or improving spaces in ways that may reduce or limit someone's ability to benefit from their privilege. When thinking about the costs of fighting for change, also consider the following.

- How might your change efforts be received by the people around you who have the most privilege?
- Might any of them resist your efforts? If so, what might their resistance look like, and could their resistance result in any social, resource, safety, or emotional costs to you?

4. **Evaluate your options.** Use the worksheet on the facing page to evaluate your options.

5. **Decide whether to make a change effort.** Time to decide how you want to move forward. After considering the pros and cons of engaging in a change effort, answer the question "Are you planning to engage in any change efforts to pursue your change goal at this time?" See the worksheet on page 162.

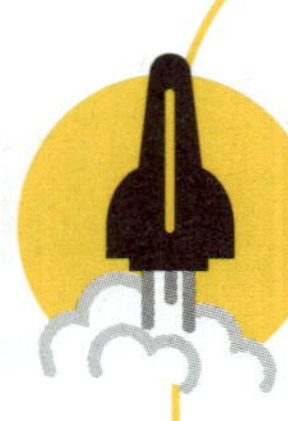

Power Up! Tips for Boosting Your Empowered Coping

This five-step process involves significant work, so it's easy to expect an immediate "payoff." Please remember that the word *effort* is a reminder to acknowledge that any decision to pursue change, correction, or improvement can still be valuable and meaningful even if it does not lead to immediate desired outcomes. You can still feel empowered even if not 100% satisfied with the outcome.

Evaluating My Options for Pursuing Change

A. List your possible actions: Select one or two change efforts you are strongly considering under "possible change efforts."

B. Complete "most helpful" column. List any reasons a change effort might be helpful. Specifically, consider whether there are any *desired* outcomes that may result from making a change effort.

C. Complete "least helpful" column. List any reasons a change effort might *not* be helpful. Specifically, consider whether there are any *undesired* outcomes that may result from making a change effort.

POSSIBLE CHANGE EFFORTS	WHAT IS *MOST HELPFUL* ABOUT THIS OPTION?	WHAT IS *LEAST HELPFUL* ABOUT THIS OPTION?
1.		
2.		

Deciding Whether to Pursue Change

A. I plan to *engage* in a change effort. If answering yes, use the table below. Describe the change effort(s) you are willing to make, describe when you plan to make these efforts, and consider ways you can cope ahead for any costs you may experience from the change efforts you make.

DESCRIBE YOUR EFFORT	WHEN DO YOU WANT TO PRACTICE?	COPE AHEAD PLAN
CHANGE EFFORT 1:		
CHANGE EFFORT 2:		
CHANGE EFFORT 3:		

B. *I do not plan to engage* in a change effort. However, if you do not think now is the best time to make a change effort, then brainstorm resilience efforts you can still engage in while in this relationship or community space.

"I don't think it's in my best interest to try a change effort at this time."	**Describe any resilience efforts you can still engage in.** (*Note:* If unsure of resilience efforts you can make, see Chapter 14 for assistance.)

Chapter 13: Recap and Reflect

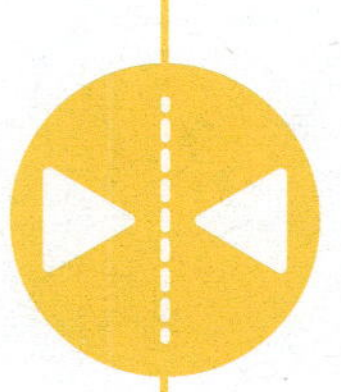

RECAP

- **Change goals** are any ideas or desires you have for changing, correcting, or improving surroundings to be less culturally stressful.
- This chapter outlined the following steps for pursuing any change goals you might have:
    1. Clarify what your change goals are.
    2. Brainstorm change efforts for pursuing these goals.
    3. Consider the costs of fighting for change.
    4. Evaluate your options (pros and cons).
    5. Decide whether to make a change effort.

REFLECT

When you choose to make a change effort (now or in the future), it's important to take time to reflect on what you've learned from this experience. Also, such reflection can help you acknowledge the ways you've made efforts to find your sense of control and to take action within your relationships and community spaces. Use the questions below to consider any important lessons learned from your change efforts.

Why was it important to you to make an effort to change, correct, or improve your culturally stressful surroundings?

Which of your personal abilities have you been able to use to make change efforts? *Note:* If you're having a hard time identifying such abilities, see the personal strengths you listed in your Who Am I? diagram in Chapter 1 (page 14).

Are there any personal abilities that you still need to improve to support your change efforts?

Have you found helpful ways to cope ahead for any costs you have incurred from engaging in change efforts?

14 How Can I Maintain Progress toward My Goals in Stressful Surroundings?

It would be amazing if we could confidently use our change efforts to make culturally stressful surroundings less stressful *and* have the assurance that doing so would lead to immediate change. Also, it would be great if we knew for sure we would be free from any unwanted costs or negative consequences of our change efforts. But, as you may know, at times life doesn't work that way. Sometimes it may be in your best interest to shift your focus away from fighting for immediate change and instead find ways to meaningfully remain within culturally stressful settings that you must continue to be in.

In this chapter, we carefully consider the word *resilience*. Can you think of times in your life when you've heard this word used? Or possibly when you've been encouraged to build your resilience? In essence, resilience is your ability to repeatedly make intentional efforts toward a valued goal despite facing difficult and challenging circumstances. This chapter will outline steps for creating a plan for making resilience efforts.

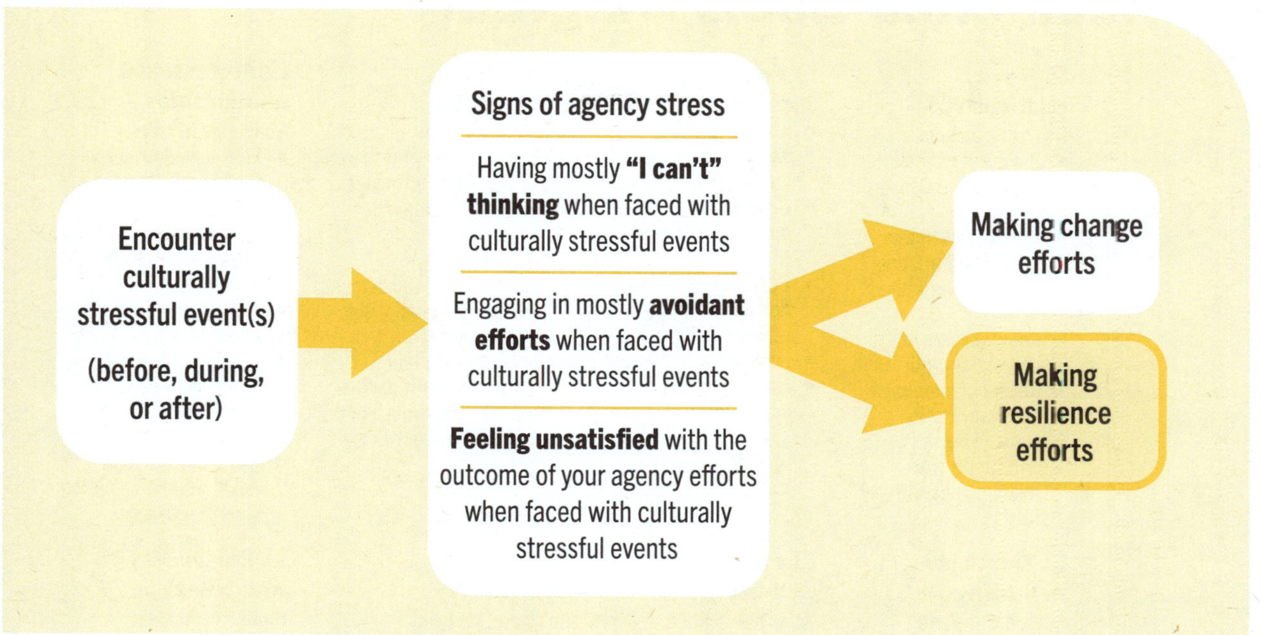

HOW TO MAKE RESILIENCE EFFORTS WHILE IN CULTURALLY STRESSFUL SPACES

The following steps will help you identify resilience efforts that you want to make while within a stressful relationship or community space. You'll also identify strategies for navigating cultural stress as you make these efforts during moments when you feel like fighting for change is not in your best interest.

1. **Identify your resilience goals.** The resilience goals you set depend on how you answer the question "What can I still accomplish or achieve while remaining within this culturally stressful setting?" You may find it helpful to brainstorm answers by categories—*relationship goals, wellness goals,* and *personal achievement goals*—that you can try to achieve both in and outside of this setting. Review examples of resilience goals you might set for yourself in the **Resilience Goals Diagram** on the next page to get your brainstorming started. Add any others that come to mind at the bottom of the lists.

2. **Brainstorm resilience efforts.** To reach any goal, it's important to brainstorm the steps toward achieving it. As you might imagine, there are many ways to prioritize and take steps toward your relationship, wellness, or achievement goals within a culturally stressful setting. Select one goal from the Resilience Goals diagram and then think of at least three options for starting (or continuing) to pursue it.

Resilience Goals Diagram

RELATIONSHIP GOALS	☐ **Family relationships** Goals can include: • Build and maintain deep connections with family • Build and maintain honest and trusting relationships with family • Communicate my boundaries with family • Respect boundaries set by my family • Have loving and supportive relationships with my family	☐ **Friendships** Goals can include: • Find people who share my interests in hobbies/fun • Build and maintain deep connections with friends • Build and maintain honest and trusting relationships • Have fun with friends • Have loving and supportive friendships	☐ **Romantic relationships** Goals can include: • Find a partner who shares my interests and values • Build and maintain deep connection with my partner • Build and maintain honest and trusting relationship with partner • Build and maintain intimacy with my partner • Build and maintain healthy communication with my partner	☐ **Professional relationships** Goals can include: • Find coworker(s) who shares my interests and values • Find coworker(s) whom I can trust is an ally at work • Work as a collaborative team member at work • Support or mentor others who want to achieve similar professional goals • Build and maintain healthy communication with coworkers
WELLNESS GOALS	☐ **Emotional well-being** Goals can include: • Mindfully notice what I am feeling • Effectively communicate my emotions • Regularly engage in soothing/relaxing activities • Practicing healthy, affirming self-talk • Being able to maintain progress toward important goals even when experiencing strong emotions	☐ **Physical well-being** Goals can include: • Get the recommended amount of nightly sleep • Create a work-life balance that promotes rest • Get consistent exercise • Maintain nutritious, balanced diet • Maintain regular check- ups with my doctor • Take medications as prescribed	☐ **Spiritual well-being** Goals can include: • Learn more about my faith • Learn more about the faith of others • Prioritize time for religious or spiritual practices • Build and maintain connection with a community that shares my faith • Allow the values and beliefs of my faith to guide my decisions in life	☐ **Community well-being** Goals can include: • Learning about different parts of my community • Providing service or volunteering to promote betterment of my community • Creating resources that can benefit my community • Building relationships with members of different communities • Participating in activism or social justice to better my community
ACHIEVEMENT GOALS	☐ **Education** Goals can include: • Find academic subjects that I really care about • Discover academic subjects that are exciting • Maintain good academic performance • Improve my academic performance • Graduate with a degree that will help my future	☐ **Job/career** Goals can include: • Find a job/career that interests me • Find a job/career that will allow me to earn an income I can live on • Maintain good job performance • Get promoted within my job/career • Create a new job/career that better suits my interests and skills	☐ **Personal growth** Goals can include: • Learn more about who I am • Learn more about my strengths and values • Set achievable goals • Observe myself achieving more of the goals I set for myself • Feel more disciplined and self-controlled in my daily life • Feel more at peace with my decisions and who I am becoming	☐ **Hobbies/fun** Goals can include: • Find recreational activities I enjoy • Prioritize regularly engaging in fun activities • Improve my knowledge and skills within my hobbies • Share my hobbies with others • Experiment with and learn about new hobbies
	Describe any other resilience goals you can try to achieve in culturally stressful settings:			

3. **Brainstorm ways to support your resilience efforts.** When faced with culturally stressful relationships and community spaces, it can be difficult to keep up your efforts toward resilience goals. With relationship stressors, you might deal with ongoing judgment or mistreatment. And community stressors can leave you feeling like you don't have the support or resources needed to achieve your goals. It's important to honor the ways cultural stress can make even the best and most strategic resilience efforts seem ineffective and pointless. That's why being thoughtful and selective in how you're going to try to achieve your goals and who you trust to support your efforts is key. The table below lists three types of supportive actions that can help you endure and navigate culturally stressful experiences as you try to reach your resilience goals—information seeking, engaging in selective energy and effort, and maintaining support networks.

Actions That Can Support Reaching Resilience Goals

Supportive actions	Examples
Information seeking *What do you feel is important to learn about your surroundings that would help you know how to best achieve your goals?*	• Learning who can be trusted with certain information before sharing more • Observing who can be reliable as a support person/system • Observing which people support and respect at least one of your ideas before sharing all of your ideas
Selective energy and effort *Based on the information you have learned about your surroundings, how much energy, time, and effort do you want to invest in achieving any goals within this space?*	• Signing up to participate in clubs/committees that support your goal • Remaining in the culturally stressful setting for only the hours you are required to be there • Volunteering for projects only when others on the project are known to be fair and kind when dividing up work responsibilities
Maintaining support networks *Which relationships do you want to invest time and energy into maintaining as you try to achieve your goals?*	• Meeting with mentors who can help you navigate the stresses within a work setting • Establishing relationships with other POCs who seem supportive and trustworthy • Scheduling hangouts with friends throughout your school day to offset the culturally stressful experiences you have around certain classmates

4. Create your resilience goal plan. Pulling together the information you gathered in the first three steps, you can now create a resilience goal plan that summarizes the efforts you intend to use to progress toward your goal. Here is where you will select the resilience efforts you want to focus on in the moment. Then you will list one or two supportive actions from step 3 that you want to take to navigate any culturally stressful experiences that may come up while pursuing your resilience goals.

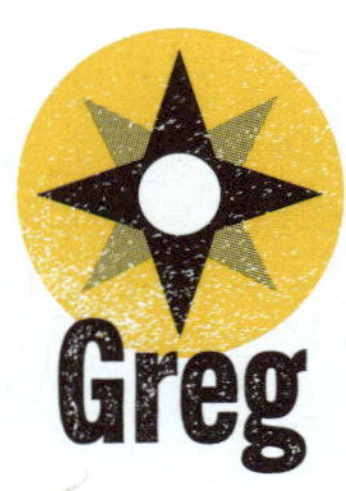

Greg's Plan for Making Resilience Efforts

Greg has had his eyes set on leaving town to attend college because he doesn't feel his community offers him the educational and career opportunities he's looking for. If you recall from Chapter 2, this is an example of a community stressor. But he recently learned that he was not awarded the scholarships he needs to attend his desired school. Now he'll have to attend the local community college and reapply for financial assistance next year. Of course, Greg is devastated by this news, so he's been using the emotional stress coping skills from Part Two of this book. He is also noticing that he's experiencing agency stress because he cannot think of any change efforts he can make to gain access to all of the educational and career opportunities he desires while remaining in his community. So Greg completed the exercises in this chapter to help him identify resilience efforts he can still make while he stays put for at least the next year.

1. Identify your resilience goals. Greg isn't quite sure what his relationship goals are, but he was able to think of some wellness and achievement goals he wants to pursue.

REFLECTION PROMPTS	RESPONSES	MY RESILIENCE GOALS AND REASONS
RELATIONSHIP GOALS *Are there any relationship goals you want to achieve within your culturally stressful surroundings?*	○ Yes ○ No ● Unsure	I can't really think about what goals I have for my relationships right now.
WELLNESS GOALS *Are there any wellness goals you want to achieve within your culturally stressful surroundings?*	● Yes ○ No ○ Unsure	I gotta keep my head on straight despite this setback. I need to make sure I am taking care of my mental health right now. But, man this is tough.
ACHIEVEMENT GOALS *Are there any achievement goals that you want to progress toward despite being in your culturally stressful surroundings?*	● Yes ○ No ○ Unsure	I want to get a high enough GPA that would allow me to qualify for any merit-based scholarships offered to students transferring from a 2-year college to a 4-year college.

2. Brainstorm resilience efforts. Greg decided to use the remainder of this worksheet to find ways to take steps toward transferring to a 4-year college.

1. I could pursue my resilience goal by . . .

attending all my classes and completing all of my homework assignments.

2. I could pursue my resilience goal by . . .

researching 4-year programs that will accept this school's credits.

3. I could pursue my resilience goal by . . .

getting a part-time job and beginning to save money for tuition at whatever 4-year college I attend—just in case I don't get a big enough scholarship.

3. Brainstorm ways to support your resilience efforts. Greg anticipates continuing to face community stressors as he pursues his goal of transferring to a 4-year school—like lacking access to needed financial resources and to peers of color who he feels are supportive of his academic pursuits. Here are some ways that Greg discovered he could use supportive actions to keep up his efforts and navigate these stressors over the next year.

	MY SUPPORTIVE ACTIONS
INFORMATION SEEKING	I could find a few campus clubs for students of color and see what their thoughts are about being at the 2-year school. I could also go to the financial aid office to get information about any options for financial aid that I missed or didn't know about while in high school.
SELECTIVE ENERGY AND EFFORT	I am not sure how much energy and effort I want to invest in activities at the community college. Maybe I can get more information about how I feel about being at this school and then revisit this supportive action.
MAINTAINING SUPPORT NETWORKS	I have a few friends I have made who are going off to 4-year colleges. Maybe I can see if they will be cool with me visiting them at their school. I can also see if there are any other students at my 2-year school who have the same goal of going to a 4-year school. Making friends with them could help me be less miserable.

4. Create your resilience goal plan. Finally, Greg was able to come up with some good ideas for pursuing his goal of transferring to a 4-year school. The worksheet below shows the steps Greg wants to prioritize toward his resilience goal.

Your resilience goal:	Transferring to a 4-year school.
What **resilience efforts** do you plan to use to help you achieve your resilience goal?	**Resilience effort 1—I plan to . . .** attend all of my classes this week. **Resilience effort 2—I plan to . . .** find a part-time job.
What **supportive actions** can you use to navigate cultural stressors as you try to achieve your resilience goal?	**Supportive action 1—I plan to . . .** use information seeking to help me learn more about different options for financial aid. **Supportive action 2—I plan to . . .** maintain support networks with my friends who are at other schools, and see what they like and dislike about their 4-year schools.

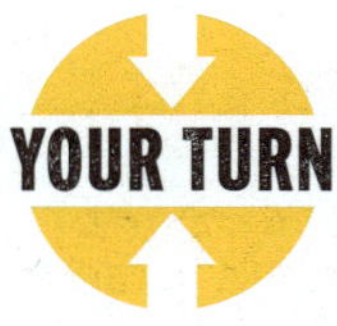

Before you get started, describe a culturally stressful event that you want to focus on for the remainder of this chapter. This can be a past, present, or anticipated event. Then follow the steps below to help you think through what engaging in resilience efforts could look like in response to that culturally stressful event.

1. Identify your resilience goals. "What do I want to achieve while remaining within my culturally stressful surroundings?" Use the worksheet on the facing page. If you have any difficulty thinking about your resilience goals, look back at the Resilience Goals Diagram on page 166.

2. Brainstorm resilience efforts. To achieve any goal it's important to brainstorm steps toward achieving it. First, pick one of your resilience goals from step 1. Then, list at least three options for pursuing your resilience goal at this moment in the worksheet on page 172.

My Resilience Goals

RESILIENCE GOALS TO CONSIDER	RESPONSES	MY RESILIENCE GOALS AND REASONS
RELATIONSHIP GOALS *Are there any relationship goals you want to achieve within your culturally stressful surroundings?*	o Yes o No o Unsure	
WELLNESS GOALS *Are there any wellness goals you want to achieve within your culturally stressful surroundings?*	o Yes o No o Unsure	
ACHIEVEMENT GOALS *Are there any achievement goals that you want to progress toward despite being in your culturally stressful surroundings?*	o Yes o No o Unsure	
Do you have any other resilience goals while remaining in the culturally stressful environment? If yes, describe them.	o Yes o No o Unsure	

My Possible Resilience Efforts

1. **I could pursue my resilience goal by . . .**

2. **I could pursue my resilience goal by . . .**

3. **I could pursue my resilience goal by . . .**

3. **Brainstorm ways to support your resilience efforts.** First, consider the ways the culturally stressful relationship or community space can make achieving your resilience goal difficult. Then use the worksheet on the facing page to help you brainstorm any supportive actions you could use to keep up your efforts and navigate cultural stress.

4. **Create your resilience goal plan.** Pulling together the information you gathered in the first three steps, you can now create a resilience goal plan. In the **My Resilience Goal Plan worksheet** on page 174, remind yourself of the resilience goal you are focusing on from step 1 by entering your goal into the lefthand column. Then, list one or two resilience efforts that you want to begin (or continue) making right now. Finally, select one or two supportive actions that you plan to use to help you achieve your resilience goal.

Possible Ways to Support My Resilience Efforts

SUPPORTIVE ACTIONS TO CONSIDER	MY SUPPORTIVE ACTIONS
INFORMATION SEEKING *What do you feel is important to learn about the relationships around you or the community space you are in that would help you pursue your goals?* *How can you go about getting this information—possibly observing others, asking specific questions, or researching certain details online?*	
SELECTIVE ENERGY AND EFFORT *Based on the information you have learned about your surroundings, how much energy, time, and effort do you want to invest in achieving any goals within this space?* *What are the pros and cons of investing more or less energy and effort within your culturally stressful surroundings?*	
MAINTAINING SUPPORT NETWORKS *Are there any relationships within or outside this space that you want to invest time and energy in maintaining and leaning on as you try to achieve your goals?* *What can you do to start and then strengthen your supportive networks?*	
Describe any other supportive actions you can engage in to navigate cultural stress as you *try to achieve* your resilience goal.	

My Resilience Goal Plan

What **resilience efforts** do you plan to use to help you achieve your resilience goal?	**Resilience effort 1—I plan to . . .** **Resilience effort 2—I plan to . . .**
What **supportive actions** can you use to navigate cultural stressors as you try to achieve your resilience goal?	**Supportive action 1—I plan to . . .** **Supportive action 2—I plan to . . .**

Chapter 14: Recap and Reflect

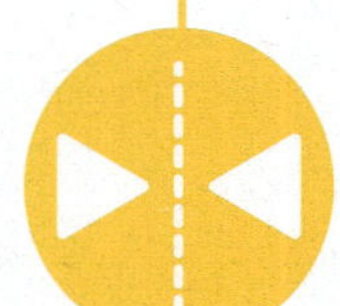

RECAP

- **Resilience goals** are meaningful goals we want to pursue while remaining within a culturally stressful environment.
- This chapter outlined the following steps for helping you pursue any resilience goals you might have.
    1. Identify your resilience goals.
    2. Brainstorm resilience efforts for pursuing these goals.
    3. Brainstorm ways to support your resilience efforts.
    4. Create a resilience goal plan.

REFLECT

When you choose to make a resilience effort (now or in the future), it's important to take time to reflect on what you've learned from this experience. Such reflection can help you acknowledge the ways you've made efforts to find your sense of control and agency within your relationships and community spaces. Use the questions below to consider any important lessons learned from your resilience efforts.

Why is it important to you to keep making efforts toward the resilience goals you selected in this chapter?

Which of your personal abilities have you been able to use to make resilience efforts? *Note:* If you're having a hard time identifying such abilities, see the personal strengths you listed in your Who Am I? diagram in Chapter 1 (page 14).

Are there any people around you who have reliably supported your resilience efforts? *Note:* This question is asking about the supportive action of maintaining support networks.

Besides maintaining support networks, what supportive actions have you found that help you navigate cultural stress and progress toward your resilience goal? *Note:* You may want to consider whether any skills in Part Two or Part Four of this workbook can also support you as you try to achieve your resilience goals.

PART THREE SUMMARY AND TAKEAWAYS

- **Agency stress** results when you struggle to know how to change, correct, improve, or endure your culturally stressful surroundings.
- In Chapter 10 you learned how to notice the moments when you're experiencing agency stress. Specifically, you learned to use the BEAT diagram as well as the My Agency Thoughts worksheet to practice **mindfulness.**
- In Chapter 11 you learned that some people can become self-critical of how they respond to culturally stressful moments. To navigate this territory (if you ever experience this), you can use **self-compassion** to show kindness and understanding toward your natural and at times unsatisfactory responses to culturally stressful events.
- Chapter 12 walked you through the two paths you can take to address agency stress: making change efforts and making resilience efforts. You had a chance to assess which path to follow, by reading Chapter 13 or Chapter 14 (or both).
- In Chapter 13 you learned that agency stress can occur when you're unsure how

to make impactful change efforts within your culturally stressful surroundings. To help you navigate this challenge, you learned how to identify and make efforts toward achieving **change goals** within culturally stressful relationships or community spaces.

- In Chapter 14 you learned that agency stress can occur when you're unsure how to maintain progress toward important goals with culturally stressful relationships or community spaces. To help you navigate this challenge, you learned how to identify and make efforts toward achieving **resilience goals** when you have to remain within culturally stressful surroundings.

TRACK YOUR AGENCY STRESS COPING

Whenever you notice yourself experiencing agency stress during a culturally stressful event, keep track of what empowered coping decisions you make to find your sense of control and agency within culturally stressful relationships or community spaces. In the **My Agency Stress Coping worksheet** on the facing page, write the date when you noticed the agency stress and then describe whether you used any coping skills from Chapter 11 (**self-compassion**), Chapter 13 (**making change efforts**), or Chapter 14 (**making resilience efforts**). Also, there is a column for any empowered coping decisions you made that do not fall into these three categories.

My Agency Stress Coping

NOTICED AGENCY STRESS	SELF-COMPASSION	MAKING CHANGE EFFORTS	MAKING RESILIENCE EFFORTS	OTHER AGENCY STRESS COPING
Date:				
Date:				
Date:				
Date:				
Date:				
Date:				

PART FOUR

How to Cope with Identity Stress

In Chapter 1, you had the opportunity to reflect on the question "Who am I?" by exploring your identities, personal strengths, interests, and values. As noted in that chapter, your surroundings can have a strong impact on your journey of self-discovery. Your relationships and community spaces can be positive and uplifting influences on who you discover yourself to be. Yet the relationship and community stressors discussed in Chapter 2 can make it hard for you as a POC to grow and maintain love and appreciation toward your racial and cultural background.

In Part Four you are going to learn about **identity stress,** which you may experience when negative and critical feedback from your surroundings makes it hard for you to experience self-love, self-confidence, and overall pride about being a member of your racial and cultural communities. First you'll practice recognizing when culturally stressful events are creating identity stress for you. Then you'll practice coping skills that help you navigate the impact of identity stress.

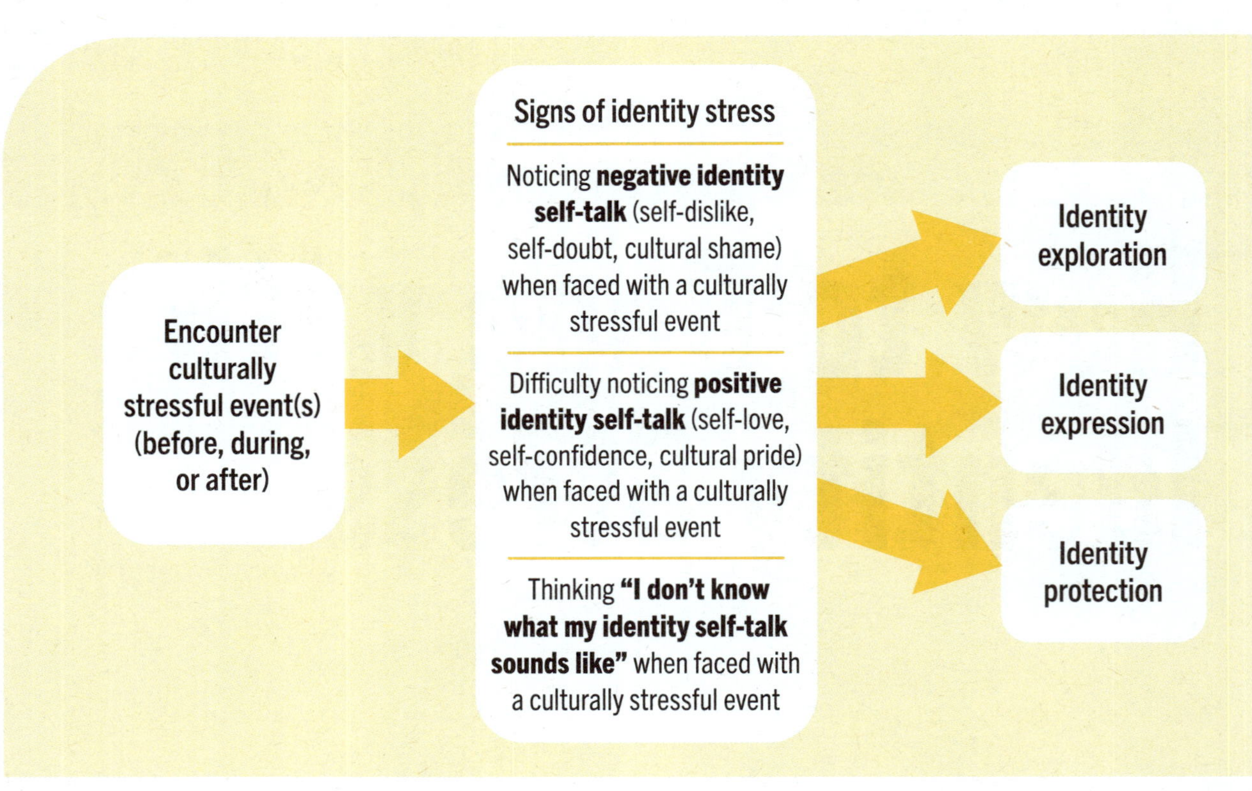

15 Noticing Identity Stress

This chapter has two main exercises: First you'll have a chance to pause and notice the moments in your daily life when you're most aware of your racial and cultural background. Sometimes these moments escape our notice among the other events of a normal busy day, so this practice is important to do. Second, you'll use the BEAT diagram (shown here) to practice noticing what types of thoughts you have about your racial and cultural background during these moments. These thoughts are often called *self-talk,* because they are the messages we give to ourselves all the time in response to what we encounter. At the end of the chapter, you'll pull together the information you gather from both exercises to determine what kinds of self-talk suggest you're struggling with identity stress.

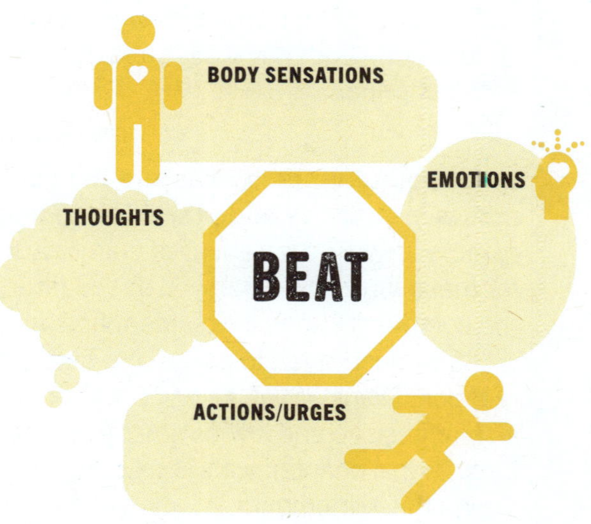

WHEN AND WHERE ARE YOU MOST AWARE OF YOUR RACIAL AND CULTURAL BACKGROUND?

There are times when your awareness of your racial and cultural background may be particularly sharp. Maybe a teacher or peer makes a race-related comment in a class. Or you come across an uplifting news story about someone within your racial and cultural community. Perhaps simply moving through parts of your neighborhood reminds you of your background. These moments may escape your attention in the rush of daily activities, especially if they are brief moments. Navigating identity stress begins with noticing these moments when they occur. So, you're first going to practice using your mindfulness skills to capture these moments as they come up in your daily life. Remember, **mindfulness** involves observing and describing your present-moment body sensations, emotions, action urges, and thoughts in response to a situation. We'll refer to the moments when you're particularly aware of your racial and cultural background as **culturally mindful moments.**

Here are the steps to identifying moments when you're most aware of your racial and cultural background.

1. **Identify the community spaces and relationships that most often prompt you to have culturally mindful moments.** Keep in mind that these moments can occur any time that your awareness of your background is heightened. They can occur during both culturally stressful events and positive moments that inspire a sense of pride.

2. **Use mindfulness to capture the culturally mindful moments you come across in your day and practice noticing your BEAT reaction to them.** One way to increase your awareness of culturally mindful moments is to set a goal to look for these moments when you spend time around any of the people or in any of the community spaces you identified in step 1. When you notice these moments, you are encouraged to pause and take a present-moment snapshot of your BEAT reaction. Doing so will help you learn how often your culturally mindful moments inspire positive and joyous emotions versus uncomfortable and painful emotions. Later in this chapter, we will take a closer look at the types of self-talk that pop up during these moments as well.

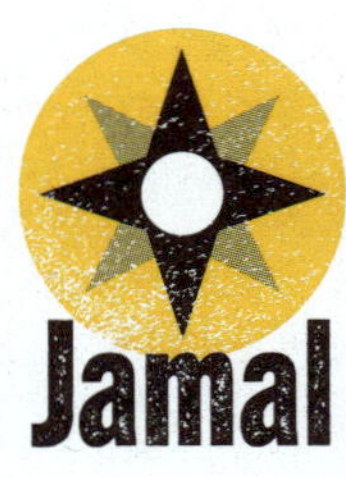

Jamal's Culturally Mindful Moments

1. Identify the community spaces and relationships that most often prompt you to have culturally mindful moments.

- **Jamal's community influences:** Jamal recalled being most aware of his Black identity when listening to hip-hop and R&B, while at his job, when attending church, and when learning of court cases that involve Black males.
- **Jamal's relationship influences:** Jamal recalled being most aware of his Black

identity when spending time with his family, when around his coworkers, and when around police officers.

2. Use mindfulness to capture the culturally mindful moments you come across in your day and practice noticing your BEAT reaction to them. Jamal set a goal of paying attention to his culturally mindful moments over the course of one week. And, on a random Wednesday while at work, Jamal walked into a staff meeting and observed that he was the only person of color in the meeting. At that moment, he noticed that he started thinking about what it's like being a Black male at his company and how he wants to show up as a Black man in this meeting. Check out his BEAT diagram to see what he noticed during this culturally mindful moment.

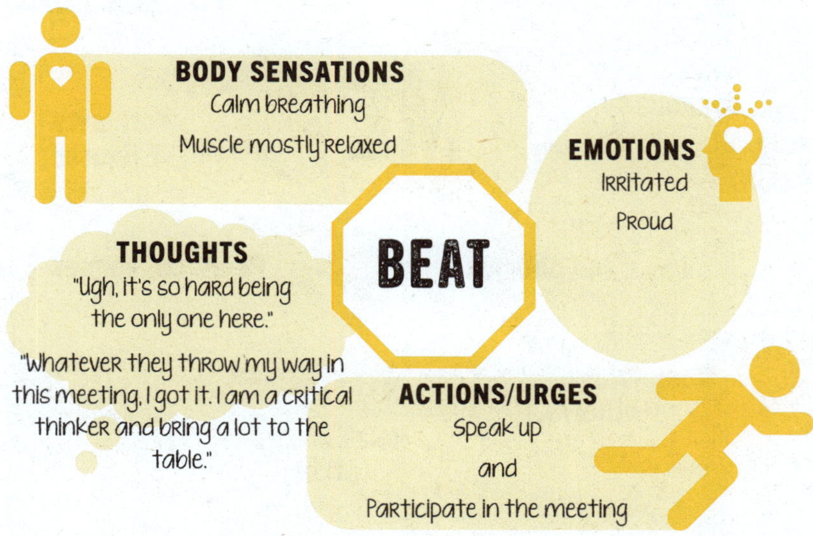

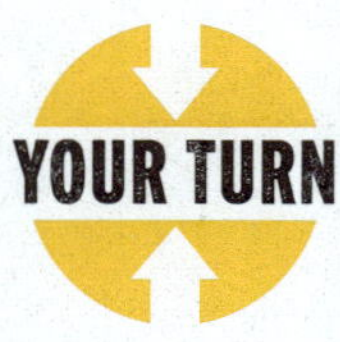

1. Identify the community spaces and relationships that most often prompt you to have culturally mindful moments. Using the diagram on the next page, *circle or highlight* each of the community spaces and relationships where you notice yourself feeling most aware of your racial and cultural background.

2. Now use mindfulness to capture the culturally mindful moments you come across in your day and practice noticing your BEAT reaction to them (use the worksheet on page 185). Over the next few days, search for at least three situations when you feel more mindfully aware of your racial and cultural background and then describe your BEAT reactions when in each situation.

My Culturally Mindful Moments

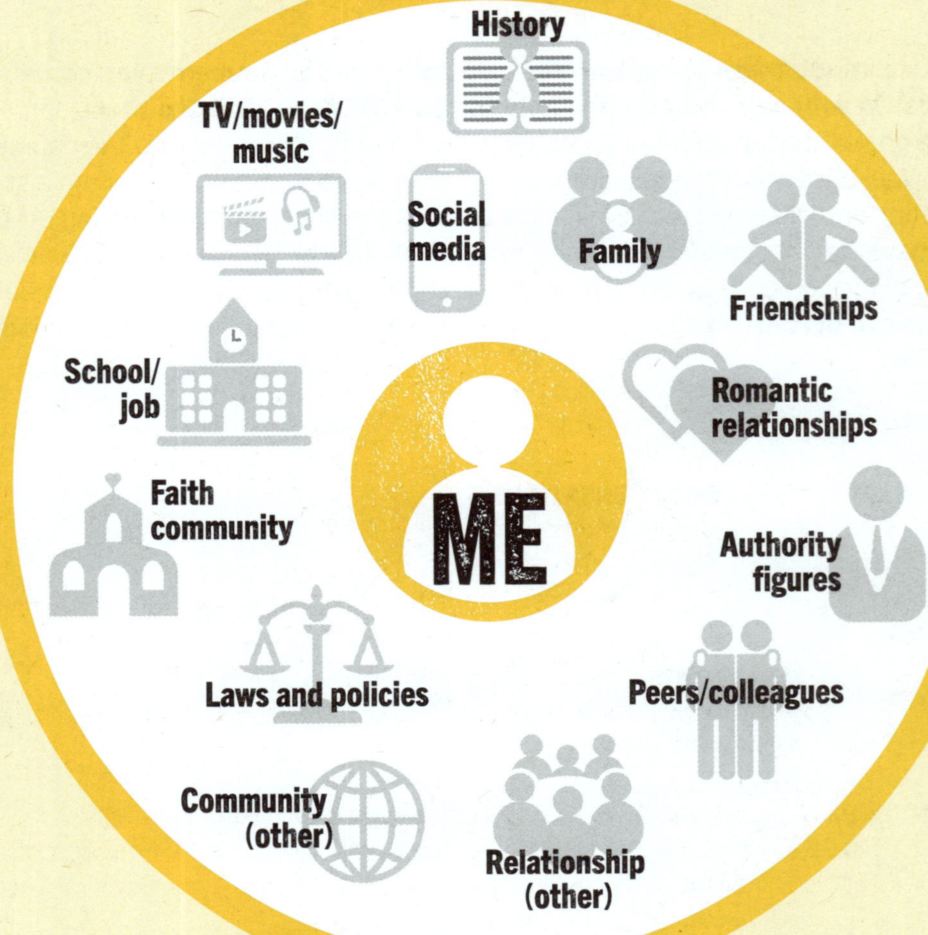

Community Influences

- **History/art:** depictions of your identity in history and art
- **TV/movies/music:** characters, plots, lyrics within any media you are exposed to
- **Social media:** messages received from followers/people followed
- **Your school/job:** performance evaluations, report cards, accessing opportunities
- **Faith community:** sermons, scriptures, prayers, people within this community
- **Laws and policies:** any laws and policies that influence the support and protection you receive
- **Other community** (any parts of community not listed)

Relationship Influences

- **Family:** immediate/extended family, adopted/chosen family, ancestors
- **Friendship:** close friends and acquaintances
- **Romantic relationships:** short-term and long-term dating partners, spouses, ex-partners, dating interests
- **Authority figures:** teachers, principals, bosses, police, politicians
- **Peers/colleagues**: people in the same community spaces as you that you do not have a close relationship with
- **Other relationship** (any relationship not listed):

My BEAT Reaction to Culturally Mindful Moments

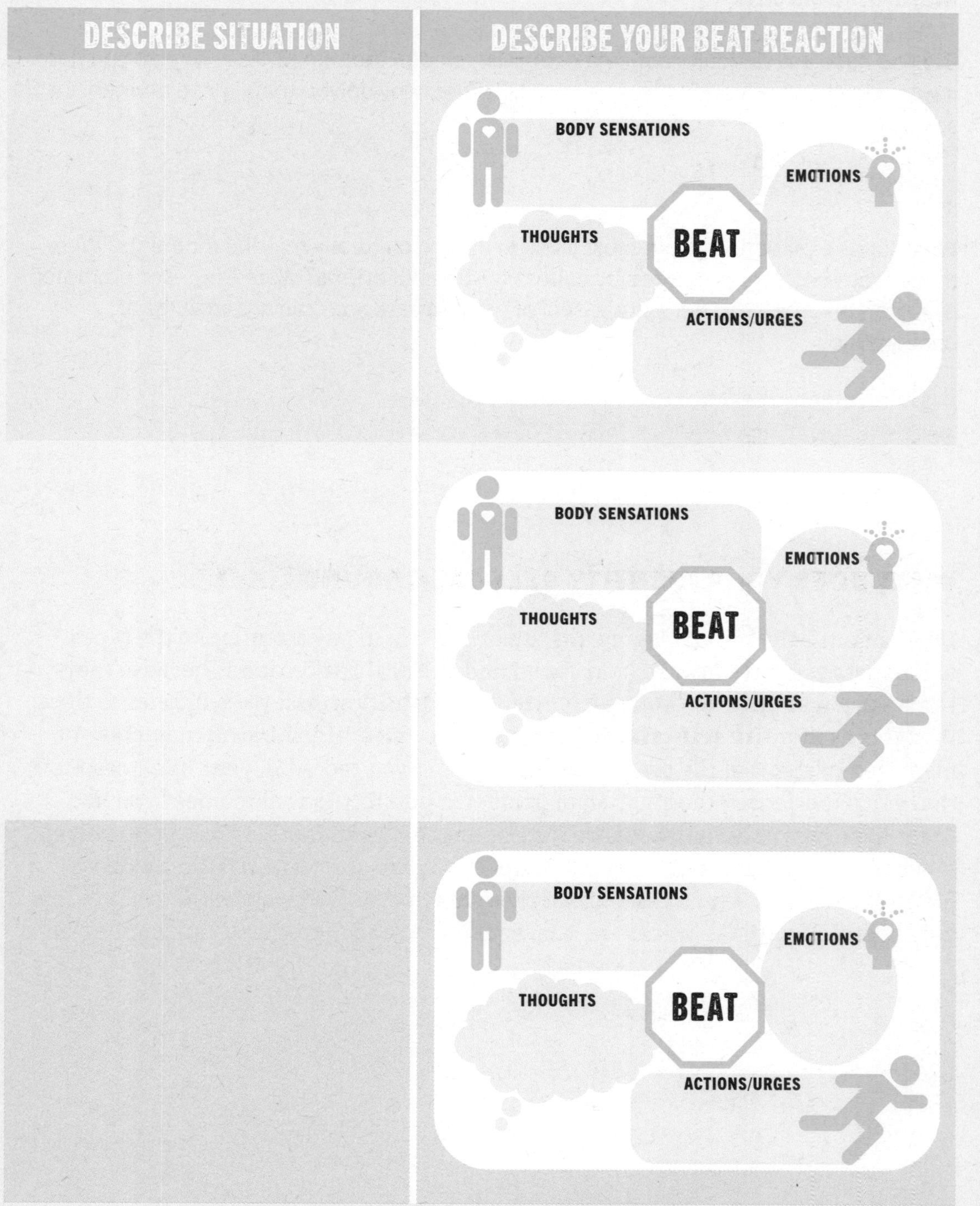

Pause and Reflect on Your BEAT Reactions to Culturally Mindful Moments

Did you have any difficulty noticing culturally mindful moments? If so, why do you think it was so difficult to notice these moments? If not, why do you think these moments were so easy to notice?

What kinds of situations were most likely to inspire culturally mindful moments? Were these moments ever prompted by culturally stressful events? Were they ever prompted by instances when you felt a great deal of pride toward your racial and cultural background?

WHAT DOES YOUR IDENTITY SELF-TALK SOUND LIKE?

During culturally mindful moments, it's important to pay attention to the types of *thoughts* you have toward your racial and cultural backgrounds because they can help you know when you're experiencing identity stress. We will refer to these thoughts as **identity self-talk.** During the three culturally mindful moments you identified in step 2 of the preceding exercise, did you record in your BEAT reaction that you experienced the emotion of pride? Or, possibly in that moment you had urges to engage or actually engaged in actions that confidently express your racial and cultural background? These BEAT reactions are often linked with **positive identity self-talk,** which can include thoughts like "It is so wonderful to share this part of myself with the world" or "I love moments like this when I can just be me."

Notably, experiencing such self-talk on a regular basis can remind you why you love and appreciate your racial and cultural background. You may also have experienced an internal tug-of-war with **negative identity self-talk,** which describes the ways you may criticize and judge your background through a lens of dislike, doubt, and shame. Such self-talk may have come up if you experienced emotions like anxiety or shame or urges to hide certain parts of your racial and cultural background during one or more of your three culturally mindful moments.

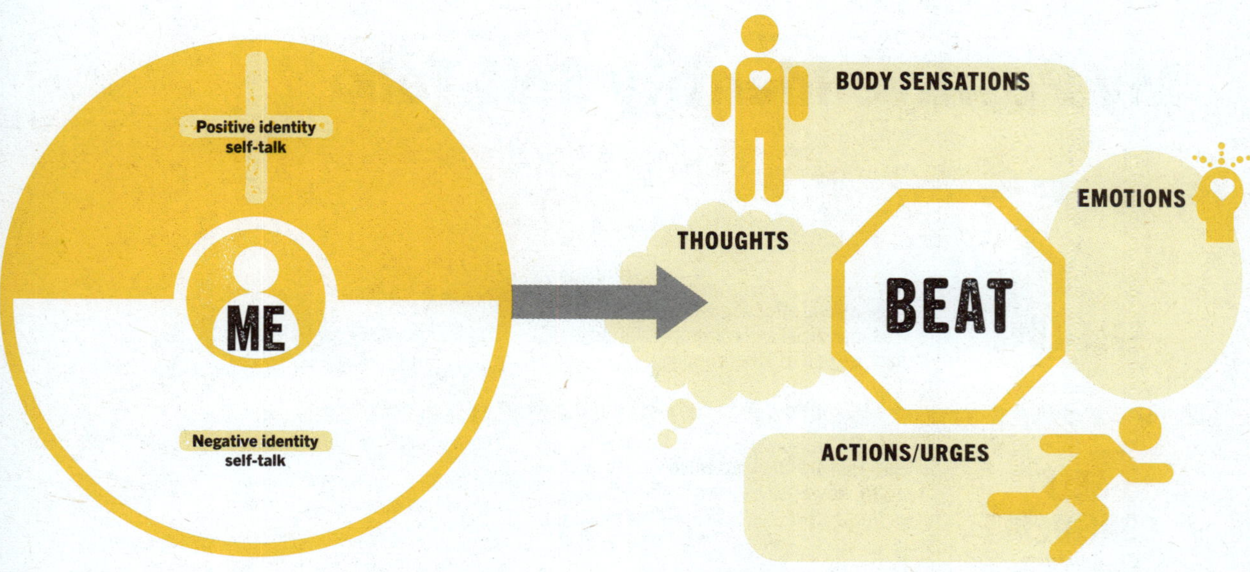

Now that you know about the two types type of identity self-talk (illustrated above), on the following pages are the steps to explore your own patterns of positive and negative identity self-talk.

1. **Notice your positive identity self-talk.** During culturally mindful moments, do you have any positive or affirming thoughts about any external attributes (like skin complexion, hair, body type) or internal attributes (like your interests, abilities, or values)? The worksheet below highlights three types of positive identity self-talk that you might have about your racial and cultural background. *Circle or highlight* any of the three types you've experienced in the lefthand column and *add any others of your own.*

My Positive Identity Self-Talk

TYPES OF SELF-TALK	DESCRIPTION	EXAMPLES
SELF-LOVE	Warm, kind, and affirming self-talk about the parts of your racial and cultural background you express or that others notice	*"My skin is beautiful."* *"I think I have really cool interests."* *"My life matters. I have meaning and purpose."*
SELF-CONFIDENCE	Self-talk that acknowledges and values your strengths, as well as believes in your ability to use these attributes to achieve meaningful goals	*"I have what it takes to get where I want to be."* *"The lessons I've learned from my community will help me get through this."* *"I am who I am. I'm gonna be me, and people will just have to accept that."*
CULTURAL PRIDE	Self-talk that expresses thankfulness and appreciation for being a member of your racial and cultural background or for being connected to other members of your community	*"I'm rooting for everyone in my community to win."* *"I am thankful to come from where I am from."* *"People from my racial and cultural community have done great things."*
List any other types of **positive identity self-talk** about your racial and cultural background.		

2. Notice your negative identity self-talk. You may also have times when the negative and critical messages from your surroundings find a way into your identity self-talk. The following worksheet highlights three types of negative identity self-talk that you might have toward your racial and cultural background when exposed to culturally stressful events. *Circle or highlight* any of the three types you've experienced in the lefthand column and *add any others of your own.*

My Negative Identity Self-Talk

TYPES OF SELF-TALK	DESCRIPTION	EXAMPLES
SELF-DISLIKE	Cold, unkind, or critical self-talk about the parts of your racial and cultural background you express or that others notice	*"I really wish I didn't look like this."* *"My interests are dumb."* *"Ugh . . . I can't stand my accent."*
SELF-DOUBT	Self-talk that ignores, criticizes, or undervalues your strengths, or that does not believe in your ability to use these self-attributes to achieve meaningful goals	*"I don't have what it takes."* *"People like me don't typically do well on these things."* *"There's no way I can show people who I really am."*
CULTURAL SHAME	Self-talk that expresses a lack of thankfulness and appreciation for being a member of your racial and cultural background or for being connected to other members of your community	*"I wish I wasn't from my racial and cultural community."* *"I don't think it's that big a deal when I see people from my community doing well."* *"I feel like people in my community are lame and make poor decisions."*
List any other types of **negative identity self-talk** about your racial and cultural background.		

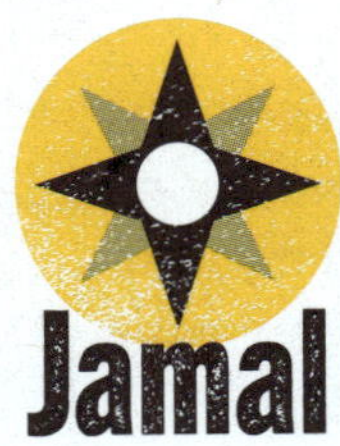

Jamal's Positive and Negative Self-Talk

Here is Jamal's **identity self-talk diagram,** where he listed the types of self-talk that he noticed come up for him during culturally mindful moments.

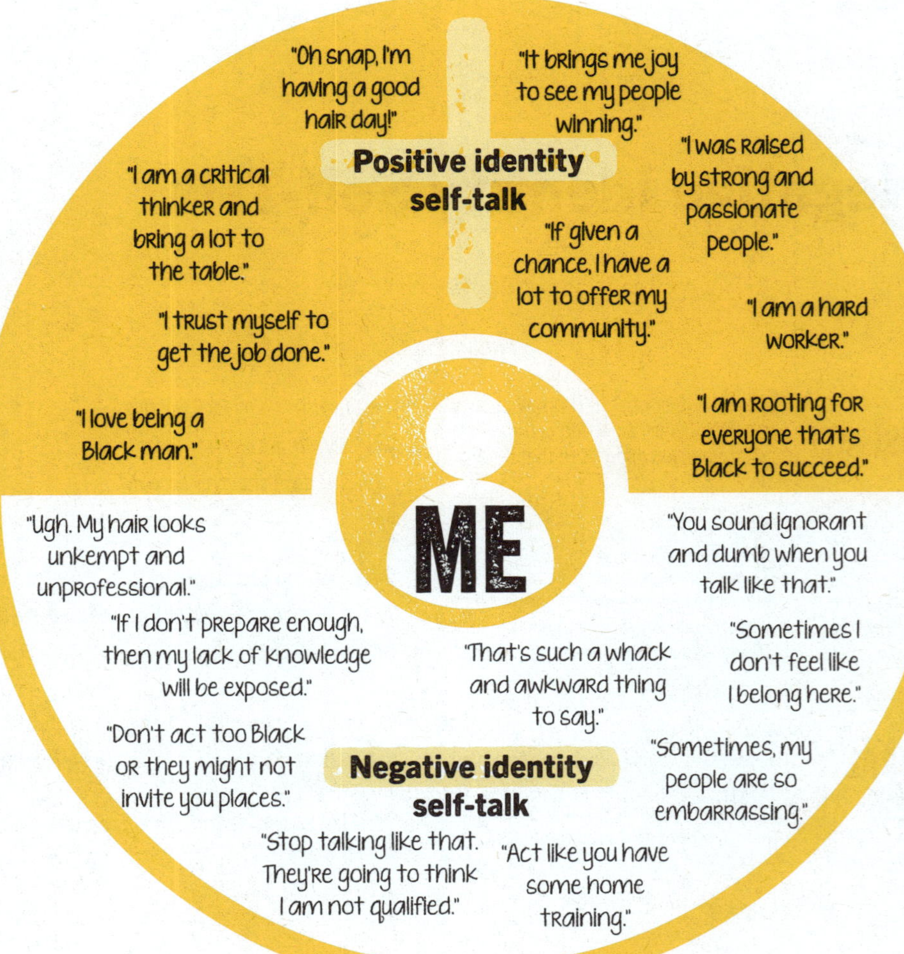

Jamal is trying to navigate and adjust to his new professional life. Jamal decided to use this exercise to build his awareness of identity self-talk at his current job, as he really hopes to boost his self-confidence and outwardly showcase his internal love and appreciation for his racial and cultural background more and more. As you can see, Jamal was able to write down examples of both types of identity self-talk. And, though he has positive identity self-talk, he was surprised to see the types of negative identity self-talk that show up more often than not at work.

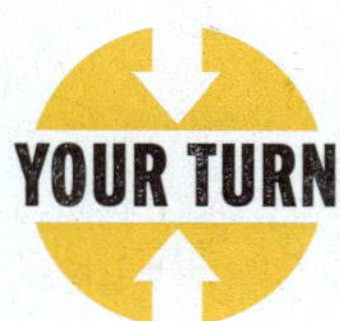

Looking back at the types of positive and negative identity self-talk that you circled in the worksheets in this chapter, fill in your own examples of each type of identity self-talk in the **My Identity Self-Talk diagram** below.

My Identity Self-Talk Diagram

Positive identity self-talk

ME

Negative identity self-talk

Pause and Reflect on Your Identity Self-Talk

Take a moment and look over your completed My Identity Self-Talk diagram. Specifically, consider the similarities and differences in how each type of identity self-talk shows up in your life and how each type impacts the ways you express your racial and cultural background.

WHAT TO THINK ABOUT	MY POSITIVE IDENTITY SELF-TALK	MY NEGATIVE IDENTITY SELF-TALK
Was it difficult to come up with examples of each type of identity self-talk?	○ Yes ○ No ○ Unsure	○ Yes ○ No ○ Unsure
Explain your answer:		
When and where do you most often notice each type of identity self-talk? Note: *Consider looking back at your My Culturally Mindful Moments earlier in the chapter*		
*What types of **body sensations** and **emotions** typically show up when you experience each type of identity self-talk?*		
How does each type of identity self-talk influence how you choose (or choose not) to express or share your racial and cultural background with others?		

HOW TO KNOW WHEN YOU'RE EXPERIENCING IDENTITY STRESS

Now that you have a better understanding of your instinctual identity self-talk, how do you know when this part of your BEAT diagram, your thoughts, might suggest you are experiencing identity stress? Here are the steps to follow.

1. Describe a culturally stressful event that you've experienced.

2. Using your BEAT diagram, record your reactions to the culturally stressful event.

3. Assess the impact the culturally stressful event had on you. Specifically, you might look for the following signs of identity stress within your BEAT reactions:

- **Presence of negative identity self-talk.** Culturally stressful events can leave POCs feeling disrespected, undervalued, unseen, or unheard. For some, such events cause them to experience self-dislike, self-doubt, or cultural shame. If you notice any of these types of identity self-talk when faced with a culturally stressful event, my hope is that a lightbulb will go off in your mind that alerts you to the identity stress you are experiencing. Acknowledging such self-talk can help you identify options for preventing these thoughts from reducing your love and appreciation toward your racial and cultural background.

- **Absence of positive identity self-talk.** Some may struggle to affirm themselves when faced with culturally stressful events. Importantly, when feeling unfairly judged, mistreated, or denied opportunities, positive identity self-talk can be an important ingredient for protecting you from the impacts of such stressful experiences. So, if you struggle to experience self-love, self-confidence, or cultural pride thoughts in the days, weeks, or months after facing culturally stressful events, this might be a sign that you're experiencing identity stress. Said differently, you could view this realization as an opportunity to find ways to boost your positive identity self-talk.

- **"I don't know what my identity self-talk sounds like."** You may have learned from completing this chapter that you haven't focused much on your identity self-talk. Possibly, you have found yourself moving through your daily life without really thinking about your racial and cultural background. And it wasn't until recently that you began the journey of trying to understand how you think and feel about this part of your identity. If this describes you in any way, I strongly recommend setting a goal of learning more about how your surroundings are impacting your ability to develop self-love, self-confidence, and cultural pride—especially in the moments that are tainted by culturally stressful events.

Now let's see how Greg used the worksheet on pages 196–197 to notice his experience with identity stress.

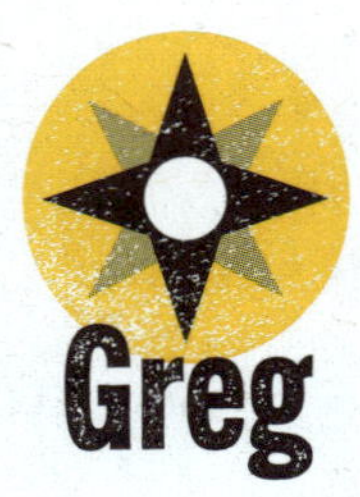

Greg's Identity Self-Talk

Greg has spent most of his time around other POCs—specifically Latinos and Black individuals. All of Greg's close friends are POCs, and most of his classmates are as well. However, Greg has often felt somewhat disconnected from other POCs—even his friends and family. His interests have always been perceived as odd and those in his community jokingly referred to them as Greg's "acting White." He's heard this so much that when at school he rarely talks about his interests. Actually, he tends to just go along with other's interests and imitates how his friend's think "real" POC's are supposed to act. The other day one of his friends saw a song he was listening to on his phone and then said, "Bro, you are so whitewashed." Greg hates hearing this, but then again sometimes questions if he really is.

1. Describe the culturally stressful situation.

Where were you?	Walking into school
Who was present?	Close friend
Describe the relationship or community stressor	Close friend told me I was whitewashed for listening to the music I listen to

2. Using your BEAT diagram, record your reactions to the culturally stressful event.

- **Describe identity self-talk.** On your BEAT diagram, describe any positive (self-love, self-confidence, cultural pride) or negative (self-dislike, self-doubt, cultural shame) identity self-talk you experienced.
- **Describe bodily sensations and emotions.** On your BEAT diagram, describe any body sensations or emotions you are experiencing in response to the culturally stressful event.
- **Describe your actions and urges.** On your BEAT diagram, describe how your identity self-talk impacted any actions or urges you experienced.

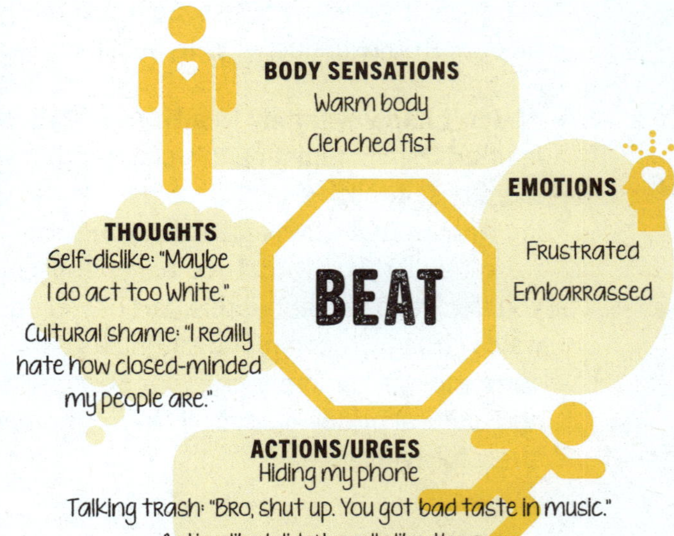

3. Describe the impact of the culturally stressful event. When looking at your BEAT diagram, do you notice yourself having any of the following?

Do you have any negative identity self-talk right now?	● Yes ○ No
Are you struggling to have positive identity self-talk right now?	● Yes ○ No
Are you unsure of your identity self-talk right now?	○ Yes ● No

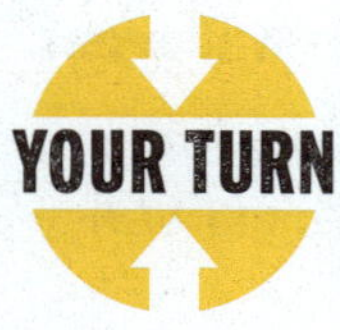

Use the **Noticing My Identity Stress** worksheet on the next page any time you are curious if you are experiencing this type of cultural stress impact.

Power Up! Tips for Boosting Your Empowered Coping

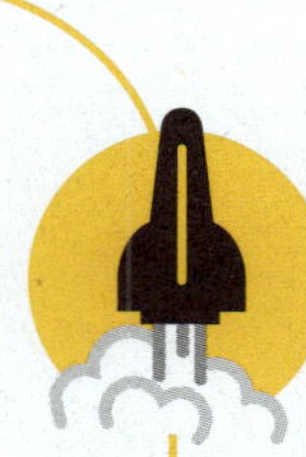

- If you answered yes to any of the three signs of identity stress, proceed to Chapter 17 to begin learning about the different coping decisions you can make when experiencing identity stress.

Noticing My Identity Stress

1. Describe the culturally stressful situation.

Where were you?	
Who was present?	
Describe the relationship or community stressor	

2. Using your BEAT diagram, record your reactions to the culturally stressful event.

- **Describe identity self-talk.** On your BEAT diagram, describe any positive (self-love, self-confidence, cultural pride) or negative (self-dislike, self-doubt, cultural shame) identity self-talk you experienced.
- **Describe bodily sensations and emotions.** On your BEAT diagram, describe any body sensations or emotions you are experiencing in response to the culturally stressful event.
- **Describe your actions and urges.** On your BEAT diagram, describe how your identity self-talk impacted any actions or urges you experienced.

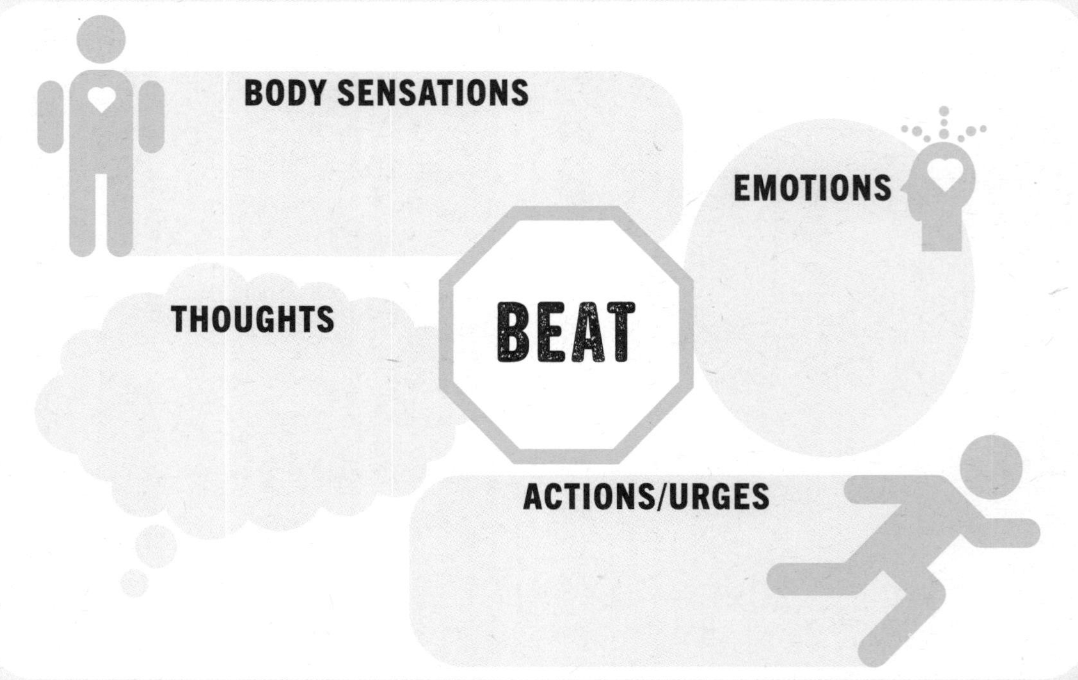

(continued)

Noticing My Identity Stress *(page 2 of 2)*

3. Describe the impact of the culturally stressful event. When looking at your BEAT diagram, do you notice yourself having any of the following?

Do you have any negative identity self-talk right now?	o Yes o No
Are you struggling to have positive identity self-talk right now?	o Yes o No
Are you unsure of your identity self-talk right now?	o Yes o No

Chapter 15: Recap and Reflect

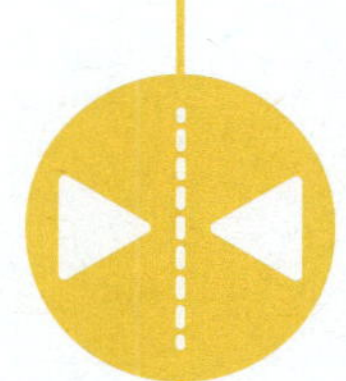

RECAP

- **Mindfulness** describes choosing to pause, observe, and describe your body sensations, emotions, action urges, and thoughts at any given moment.
- In this chapter, you learned to use the **BEAT diagram** to help you observe when you're experiencing identity stress.
- Specifically, identity stress describes when your BEAT diagram includes negative identity self-talk, an absence of positive identity self-talk, or feeling unsure what your identity self-talk sounds like.

REFLECT

Now that you have learned about this type of cultural stress impact, take a few moments to reflect on what your identity stress looks and feels like.

What types of culturally stressful events most often trigger identity stress for you?

Did you notice any particular body sensations or emotions that also occur when experiencing identity stress?

Do you ever criticize or judge yourself for having negative identity self-talk in response to a culturally stressful event? If so, what does your self-criticism or self-judgment sound like?

16 How Can I Show Kindness and Understanding toward My Identity Stress?

You just learned that identity stress is defined by struggling to express, internally and outwardly, self-love, self-confidence, and cultural pride. Why do we struggle with this? When an event is culturally stressful, it's often communicating **social messages** in the form of stereotypes, judgments, and acts of discrimination. Unfortunately, as shown in the diagram below, these social messages have a way of influencing how we think about our racial and cultural background. In this chapter, you will learn what social messages are having the greatest influence on your identity self-talk.

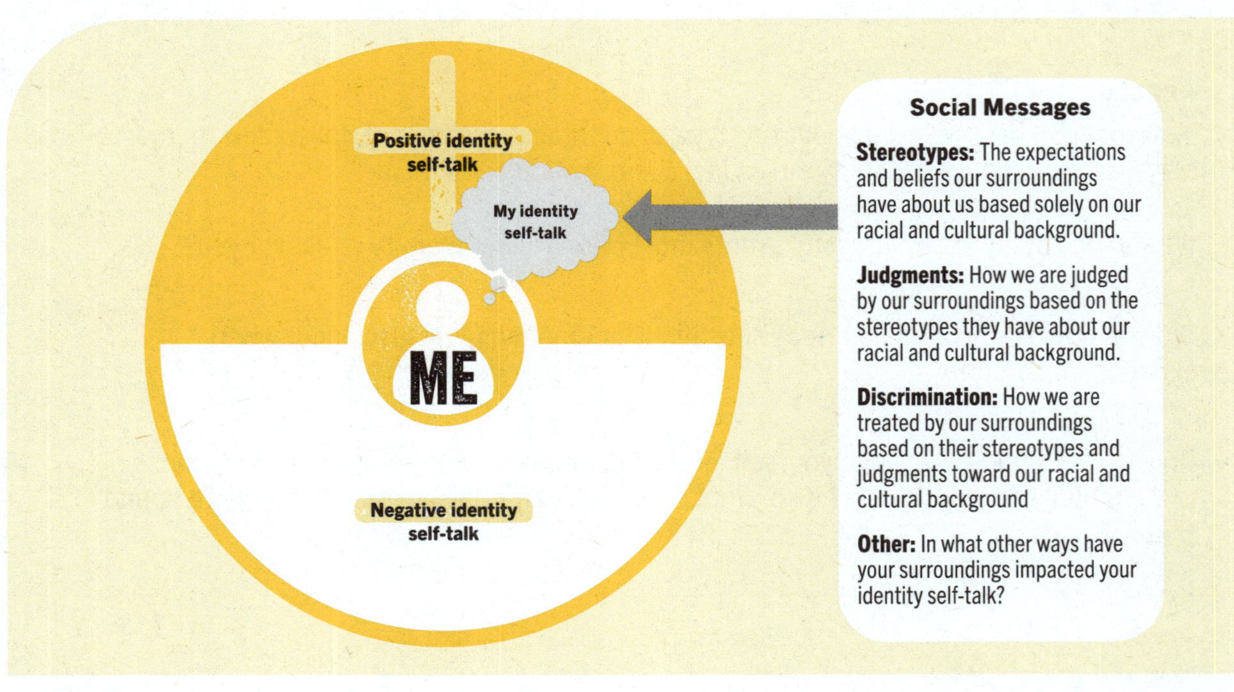

WHAT ARE SOCIAL MESSAGES?

Let's start by developing a good understanding of these terms: *stereotypes, judgments,* and *discrimination.* As shown in the diagram, we can define *stereotypes* as the expectations and beliefs used to categorize people based on their shared characteristics. Based on our stereotypes about racial and cultural groups, we all develop judgments, or quick interpretations or feelings toward people—essentially swiftly labeling someone as "good" or "bad," "likeable" or "unlikeable," or even "safe" or "dangerous" based solely on our beliefs and assumptions about their group. Finally, these stereotypes and judgments influence how we treat people of specific racial and cultural backgrounds—referred to as discrimination. Importantly, stereotypes, judgments, and acts of discrimination can become problematic and hurtful when inaccurate stereotypes are spread, when these stereotypes are not updated or changed upon meeting someone who does not fit the stereotype, or when stereotypes and judgments lead to harmful, unfair acts toward someone. Honestly, it's important that we all, regardless of our racial and cultural background, educate ourselves about our own stereotypes and judgments and remain mindful of how we treat others to avoid spreading hurtful social messages ourselves.

But, as you may have already experienced, many people and community spaces have not taken the time to examine how their stereotypes, judgments, and discriminatory actions are influencing POCs. This is one of the reasons POCs continue to be exposed to culturally stressful events. Unfortunately, this leaves you tasked with learning to build love and appreciation toward your racial and cultural background while trying to navigate the impact of the hurtful (and sometimes confusing) social messages you receive.

WHAT SOCIAL MESSAGES HAVE IMPACTED YOUR IDENTITY SELF-TALK?

When you think about stereotypes, judgments, or discrimination, your mind probably goes immediately to the negative content spread about POCs and the hurtful ways POCs have been treated. This makes sense. But there are stereotypes that we could call *positive* as well as the negative ones.

POSITIVE SOCIAL MESSAGES

Imagine a Black kid who transfers to a new school. He's in a gym class where the activity of the day is playing basketball. His peers, knowing nothing about him except for his race and gender, assume he must be athletic. Because being athletic in this case is considered a good and desirable characteristic, his classmates initially judge and treat him favorably: He's one of the first picked for a team. The sequence of social messages connected with this initial stereotype is shown in the Positive Stereotypes table.

Positive Stereotypes

Social message type	Definition	Social message example
Positive stereotypes	Beliefs or assumptions about someone's abilities, interests, or character traits based solely on their racial and cultural background	All Black people are athletic.
Judgments	Interpretations and attitudes directed at someone based on stereotypes held about someone's racial and cultural background	Being athletic is a "good" and "desirable" ability in gym class.
Discrimination	Being treated differently or given an opportunity due to the stereotypes and judgments held about someone's racial and cultural background	Black people are picked before anyone else when they are seen as athletic.

In this example, the positive stereotype held by the new kid's classmates and their associated judgment and discrimination led to social messages that would seem *positive and uplifting.* I mean, it can't be that bad to receive positive attention because someone assumes you have certain desirable traits, abilities, or interests, right? But what if these beliefs are inaccurate about this student? Have you ever been offered opportunities that don't line up with your interests, abilities, or values? If so, you may have felt like others were putting you into a narrow box—essentially communicating you will be seen as important, valued, and "cool" *only* if you fit within the beliefs and expectations that your surroundings have about your racial and cultural background. Such messages can get in the way of your ability to grow and maintain your self-love, self-confidence, and cultural pride. You could end up disliking parts of yourself or struggling to confidently express your true qualities if you can't (or don't want to) live up to the "positive" stereotypes communicated to you. That's why *positive* is in quotation marks here—these stereotypes sometimes do not lead to proud and enjoyable experiences.

Remember Greg? His friends' stereotypes about Latine culture contributed to Greg's identity stress. Essentially, his friends communicated that only certain interests make someone a "true Latino," and any interests outside of this box mean that Greg is "acting White" or is "whitewashed." Importantly, Greg's story highlights that identity stress can be caused by the social messages we receive from people who look like us and who are from our racial and cultural communities. At best, his friends may see their statements as trying to help Greg be more like them—you know, be more accepted and liked. Or, possibly, they see it as harmless joking and fun. We know, however, that they were hurtful to Greg and that these social messages made it hard for Greg to have self-loving thoughts toward his true interests while maintaining a sense of cultural pride toward his racial and cultural background.

Pause and Reflect on the Existence and Impact of Positive Stereotypes

In the **Positive Social Messages I Have Encountered worksheet** (page 202), list some of the positive stereotypes that exist about your racial and cultural background. Examples of such stereotypes include "Black people should be great dancers," "true Latinos speak fluent Spanish and love spicy foods," or "all Asian Americans are studious and smart." Then think about the judgments and acts of discrimination that have been associated with these stereotypes. Remember, these are the stereotypes that occur *both inside and outside* of your racial and cultural community. Finally, reflect on the impact of these social messages on your identity self-talk.

Power Up! Tips for Boosting Your Empowered Coping

Calling in your workbook navigators: You may find it helpful to complete this worksheet on page 202 with one of your workbook navigators who is familiar with the social messages often experienced by your community.

NEGATIVE SOCIAL MESSAGES

Stereotypes can also expose us to *negative, critical, and hurtful* messages about our racial and cultural background. For example, in the months immediately following the start of the COVID-19 pandemic, there was a growing **negative stereotype** that people appearing to have an Asian background were responsible for the start of the pandemic. Such beliefs, unfortunately, triggered very negative judgments toward members of the Asian community, which led to increased discrimination toward them, including senseless and unprovoked acts of violence. For many, these

Positive Social Messages I Have Encountered

SOCIAL MESSAGE TYPE	REFLECTION QUESTION	PERSONAL EXAMPLES
POSITIVE STEREOTYPES	What positive or desired traits, abilities, or interests do others (including those within your community) often expect people within your racial and cultural background to have?	
JUDGMENTS	How do people typically judge or feel toward these stereotypes?	
DISCRIMINATION	How have these positive stereotypes and their judgments influenced how you (or people within community) have been treated?	

REFLECT	RESPONSE	EXPLANATION
Have any of these social messages greatly impacted your ability to experience self-love, self-confidence, or cultural pride?	○ Yes ○ No ○ Somewhat	

painful and scary experiences were reminders of a long-standing stereotype about Asian people in the United States: "All Asians are foreigners." No matter how many generations of Asian families have been in the United States or how much they've contributed to their communities, these hurtful incidences communicated that "Asian people are not safe, protected, or valued members of their communities." The Negative Stereotypes table summarizes the social messages that Asian individuals could have gotten from these culturally stressful events.

Negative Stereotypes

Social message type	Definition	Social message example
Negative stereotypes	Negative and hurtful beliefs or assumptions about someone's abilities, interests, or character traits based solely on their racial and cultural background	"All Asian people are to blame for COVID-19."
Judgments	Interpretations and attitudes directed at someone based on stereotypes held about someone's racial and cultural background	Being Asian will be met with anger, rage, and disgust.
Discrimination	Culturally stressful events that include being mistreated or denied opportunities due to the stereotypes and judgments held about someone's racial and cultural background	Being Asian can cause me to be violently attacked.

Importantly, negative stereotypes can be rooted in beliefs that have been held for decades ("All Asians are foreigners"), and these stereotypes can be triggered by current events ("All Asians are to blame for COVID-19"). When such hurtful stereotypes create culturally stressful events, those impacted can find it difficult to grow and maintain self-love, self-confidence, and cultural pride.

We've seen this throughout Amia's story. Historical events like the terrorist attacks on 9/11 continue to spread negative and hurtful beliefs about the Muslim community, and many immigrants continue to be judged unjustly as outsiders and mistreated in ways that cause them to feel unwelcome within their communities. Amia feels "othered" by her classmates and even her teacher, among others.

Pause and Reflect on the Existence and Impact of Negative Stereotypes

In the Negative Social Messages I Have Encountered worksheet (on the facing page), list some of the negative stereotypes that exist about your racial and cultural background. Some examples include "all Black people are lazy and dangerous," "darker skin complexions are not as pretty as lighter skin complexions," or "all Latinos are immigrants who are trying to steal jobs from Americans." Then think about the judgments and acts of discrimination that have been associated with these stereotypes. Remember, these are the negative stereotypes that occur *both inside and outside* of your racial and cultural community. Finally, reflect on how these social messages impact your identity self-talk.

Power Up! Tips for Boosting Your Empowered Coping

Calling in your workbook navigators: You may find it helpful to complete the worksheet on the facing page with one of your workbook navigators who is familiar with the social messages experienced by your community.

In summary, our identity self-talk rarely comes out of the blue. In some way, shape, or form, our surroundings are planting seeds that sometimes cause our negative identity self-talk to grow. So what can you do when social messages toward your racial and cultural background negatively impact your thoughts and feelings about yourself?

HOW TO SHOW UNDERSTANDING TOWARD YOUR IDENTITY SELF-TALK

You may have a variety of ways of coping with the ways social messages negatively influence your thoughts and feelings about yourself. But the following exercise can help you build an *empowered* coping skill. These three steps will help you practice self-compassion when experiencing negative identity self-talk. As a refresher, this skill describes your efforts to show kindness and understanding toward your BEAT reactions.

Negative Social Messages I Have Encountered

SOCIAL MESSAGE TYPE	REFLECTION QUESTION	PERSONAL EXAMPLES
NEGATIVE STEREOTYPES	What negative or hurtful characteristics, traits, abilities, or interests do others (including those within your community) often associate with your racial and cultural background?	
JUDGMENTS	How do people typically judge or feel toward these stereotypes?	
DISCRIMINATION	How have these negative stereotypes influenced how you (and people within your community) have been treated?	
REFLECT	**RESPONSE**	**EXPLANATION**
Have any of these social messages greatly impacted your ability to experience self-love, self-confidence, or cultural pride?	o Yes o No o Somewhat	

1. **Catch your identity self-talk.** Even when we do our best to grow our self-love, self-confidence, and cultural pride, culturally stressful events have a way of planting seeds of dislike, doubt, and shame. This doesn't necessarily mean you don't like yourself or your background. It can just mean you're human and trying to figure out the tough task of loving yourself within surroundings that sometimes make doing so difficult. To show kindness and understanding toward yourself, you first acknowledge the types of identity self-talk you're experiencing.

2. **Notice the social messages around you.** It's hard to be on constant watch for all the social messages we are exposed to. So, there will be times when you overlook or ignore how certain social messages you're receiving are impacting your identity self-talk. You may, in fact, even criticize yourself for not loving yourself and your background more. When you notice negative identity self-talk, it can be helpful to take a step back and try to answer the question "Are there any hurtful or inaccurate social messages from my surroundings that are making it hard for me to love and appreciate being me in this moment?" Use the questions below to help you acknowledge which social messages are having the greatest impact on your positive or negative identity self-talk.

   - Are you aware of any **positive** or **negative stereotypes** about your racial and cultural background that are influencing your identity self-talk in this moment?
   - Are you aware of any affirming or hurtful **judgments** directed at you or your racial and cultural community that are influencing your identity self-talk in this moment?
   - Are you aware of any acts of **discrimination** directed at you or your racial and cultural community that are influencing your identity self-talk in this moment?
   - Are there any other messages that are influencing your identity self-talk in this moment?

3. **Compassionately show understanding.** The next step is to try to make sense of all this by lovingly stating to yourself what you had hoped your identity self-talk would be, what made your hopes difficult to achieve when faced with this event, and where you want to go from here.

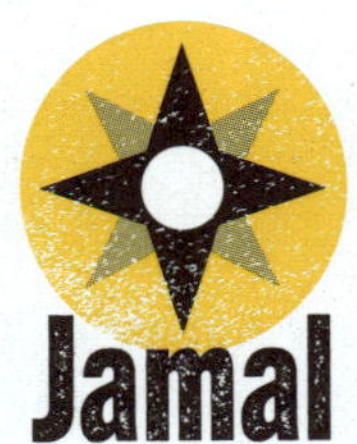

Jamal's Efforts to Show Understanding toward His Identity Stress

Before you try practicing each step, let's see how Jamal tried to turn up the volume on his compassionate narrator when he noticed lingering negative identity self-talk.

As a Black man who has spent time in mostly White academic spaces, Jamal has heard his fair share of questionable comments about his intellectual abilities from peers and teachers: "Wow, Jamal, you are so articulate," "I didn't expect you to be so smart . . . very impressive," or "You must be cheating or something. . . . How did you get a higher score on that test than I did?" While expressed in a positive or encouraging way, these comments have always felt confusing to Jamal. And, over time, he has noticed himself having a lot of self-doubting thoughts when in social spaces where these comments have been expressed—often asking himself, "Am I naturally smart, or am I just a hard worker?" This question continues to impact him even though he is no longer a student. The other day he was preparing for a presentation and couldn't get the thoughts of "I haven't done enough to prepare" and "They're going to think I'm unqualified" out of his mind. He completed this exercise to help him practice self-compassion toward these examples of negative identity self-talk.

1. **Catch your identity self-talk.** In Chapter 15, you saw Jamal's identity self-talk diagram (see page 190). Now Jamal uses this diagram to notice how social messages were impacting two examples of negative identity self-talk that came up before he made his presentation—specifically, "I haven't done enough to prepare" and "They're going to think I'm unqualified."

2. **Notice the social messages around you.** In the diagram at the top of the next page, Jamal focused on the stereotypes, judgments, and acts of discrimination that seem most related to his negative identity self-talk before his presentation. Of course, acknowledging these social messages doesn't make his identity self-talk go away or make him significantly less impacted by the presence of these thoughts. Instead, his goal is to better understand what exactly makes these thoughts come up for him before his presentation.

3. **Compassionately show understanding.** Jamal already kind of knew that he'd encountered social messages that made him feel as if he needed to be extra-prepared and to "prove" he was qualified for the work he was doing. But intentionally and explicitly reminding himself of these external influences allowed him to express kindness and compassion toward his self-doubts. For Jamal, and probably for you, it can be hard to remember to continue searching for opportunities to boost self-love and self-confident thoughts when faced with doubters and skeptics. Sometimes self-doubting thoughts seem so loud and distracting! Here's how Jamal responded to the prompts.

I would like to have this type of identity self-talk: I want to have confident thoughts about what I bring to the table at work.

However, in this situation, I noticed that my identity self-talk sounded like: I am having self-doubting thoughts that I am not prepared and I am not qualified.

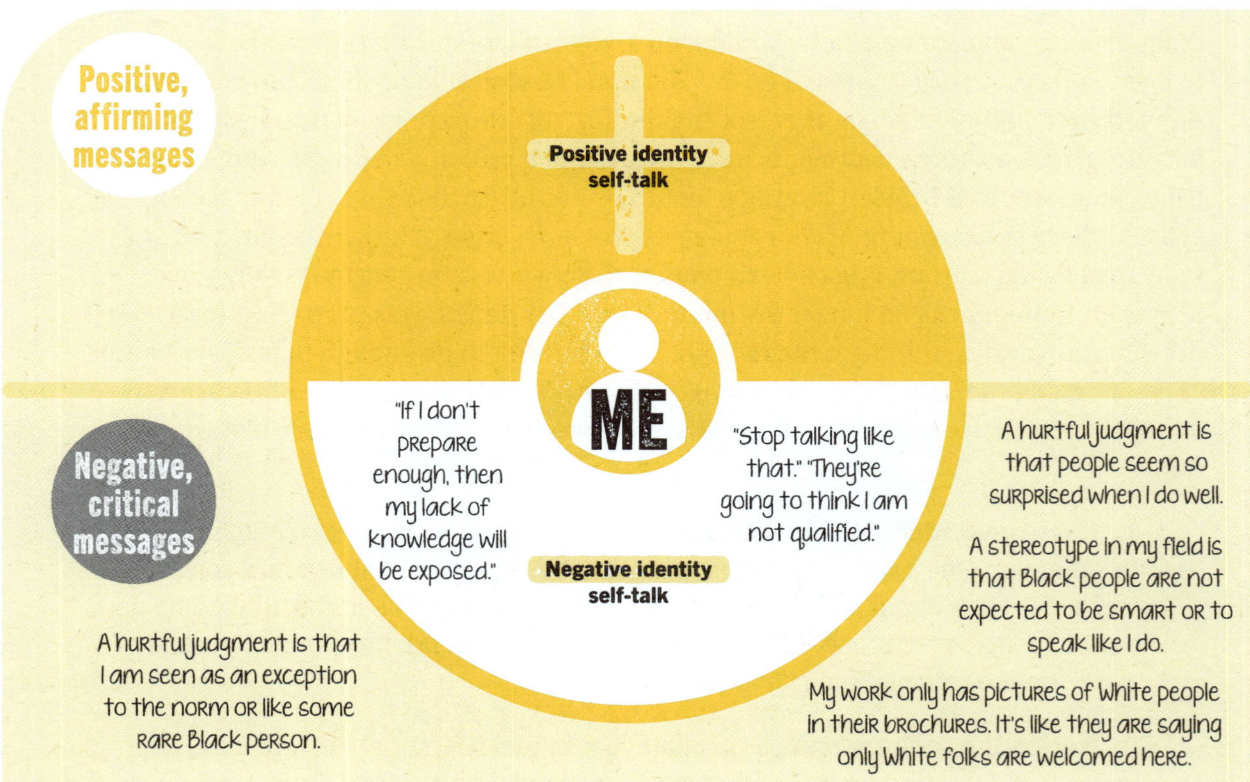

In this situation, these social messages made it hard for me to have self-love, self-confidence, or cultural pride because: I think my past experiences with people expecting less from me is making it hard for me to have more confidence right now.

It *makes sense* that these social messages would impact my identity self-talk in this way because: When I am reminded of these messages, I feel like I have to constantly prove myself. I just feel like if I have one off day, I won't be given the benefit of the doubt. I guess it makes sense that I would want to be very, very, very prepared because I feel like the stakes are so high for people who look like me.

Moving forward, I hope for myself that I will: be able to believe in myself and my capabilities even when I think people don't expect me to do well.

Moving forward, I will try to boost my self-love, self-confidence, and cultural pride by: I guess I just have to keep grinding and giving myself credit when I make progress toward my goals at work.

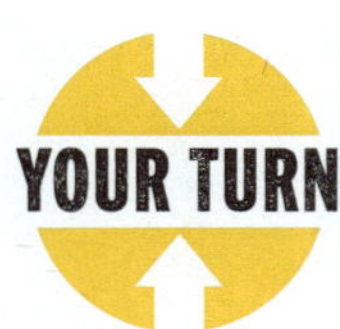

Use the steps below to help you turn up the volume on your compassionate narrator any time you face identity stress, especially in moments when you feel critical of any negative identity self-talk you're having.

1. **Catch your identity self-talk.** In the **Positive and Negative Social Messages Connected with My Identity Self-Talk diagram** below, describe any positive or negative identity self-talk you're having when faced with a culturally stressful event in the center of the diagram.

2. **Notice the social messages around you.** Next, in the diagram below, describe any positive, affirming or negative, and critical social messages that seem connected with your identity self-talk.

Positive and Negative Social Messages Connected with My Identity Self-Talk

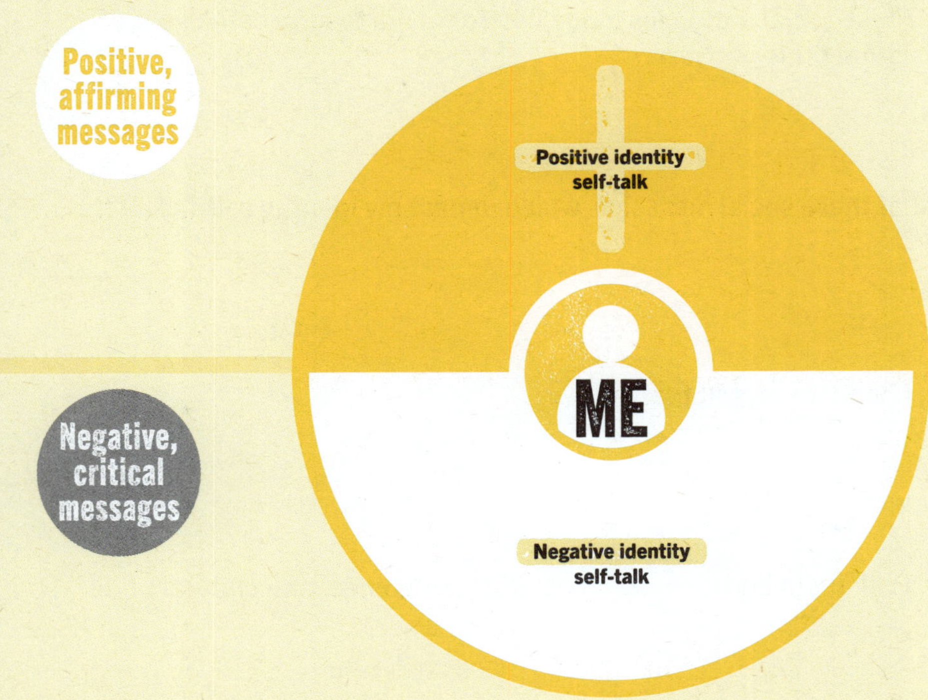

3. **Compassionately show understanding.** Try to show understanding toward your identity self-talk by completing the sentences in the worksheet below.

Compassionately Understanding My Identity Self-Talk

Typically, I like to have this type of identity self-talk:

However, in this situation, I noticed that my identity self-talk sounded like:

In this situation, these social messages made it hard for me to have self-love, self-confidence, or cultural pride because:

It makes sense that these social messages would impact my identity self-talk in this way because:

Moving forward, I hope for myself that I will:

Moving forward, I will try to boost my self-love, self-confidence, and cultural pride by:

Power Up! Tips for Boosting Your Empowered Coping
Wait, what if self-compassion doesn't work for me at first?

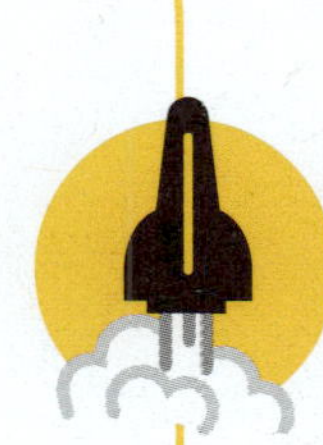

- **Compassionately respond to your emotions first.** If you've started to notice any strong and uncomfortable emotions attached to your negative identity self-talk, you may want to look back at the emotional stress coping skills in Part Two before diving into the three steps in this exercise. Sometimes the kindest and most understanding response to your BEAT reaction is to honor the reality of your emotional pain and ride the wave of discomfort first.
- **Patience and practice.** As discussed in Chapters 5 and 11, growing kindness and understanding will likely take time. Self-compassion includes giving yourself that time to practice. The self-compassion skills you develop will hopefully help you more effectively practice the remaining coping skills discussed in Part Four.
- **Start small.** When you feel ready to take a closer look at your negative identity self-talk, start with setting small goals. Possibly, set a goal to become more curious about the social messages around you and try to discuss your observations with your workbook navigators. Then, as you become more familiar with these social messages, you can try to use the sentence starters in step 3 to practice self-compassion.

Chapter 16: Recap and Reflect

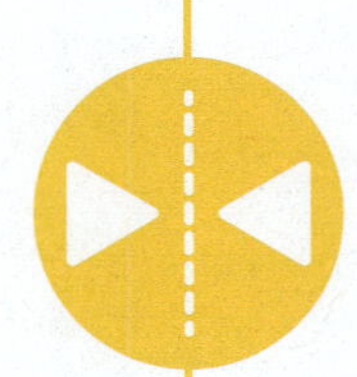

RECAP

- In Chapter 5, you learned that **self-compassion** means showing kindness and understanding toward the body sensations, emotions, action urges, and thoughts (BEAT) you're experiencing in any given moment.
- Also, you learned that developing and growing your self-compassionate narrator will help you more effectively cope with and heal from culturally stressful situations.
- One way to practice self-compassion when you have negative identity self-talk is to follow these steps:
  - Notice any negative identity self-talk.
  - Reflect on the ways social messages may impact your identity self-talk.
  - Compassionately show understanding toward the identity self-talk you are having in that moment.

REFLECT

Before moving forward, take a moment to think about what you learned about self-compassion and how you hope this skill can help you cope with identity stress. To do so, answer the questions below.

Calling in your workbook navigators: You may find it helpful to review your answers to these questions with your workbook navigators. The stereotypes, judgments, and acts of discrimination that have had the greatest impact on their self-talk can shed light on your own experiences. And you might learn additional ways to show yourself kindness and understanding when social messages are negatively impacting how you see yourself.

What does *self-compassion* mean to you, and how can it be helpful when experiencing identity stress?

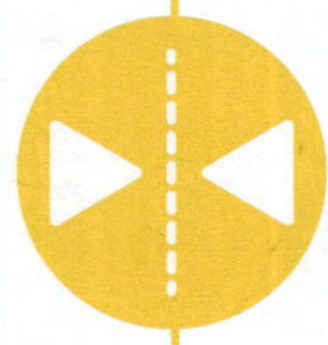

In addition to what you learned in this chapter, are there any other ways that you have learned to show kindness and understanding toward your negative identity self-talk?

How can practicing *self-compassion* enhance your ability to cope with any identity stress you experience moving forward?

17 My Identity Stress Coping Assessment

What does empowered coping for identity stress look like? You might think of it as having an offensive and a defensive game plan, as in many competitive team sports. You need coping skills to help you *increase* the love, pride, and appreciation you have toward your racial and cultural background—your offensive coping decisions. And you need coping skills that help you *protect* yourself from any social messages that limit the growth of any positive and uplifting thoughts and feelings you have toward your background—your defensive coping decisions. In this chapter, you'll follow a few steps to help you identify how you have already attempted to build and protect your self-love, self-confidence, and cultural pride when faced with culturally stressful events. Also, you will learn about opportunities for growing your ability to cope with identity stress.

HOW TO USE THE IDENTITY STRESS COPING DIAGRAM

To help you strengthen your coping skills for experiences of identity stress, you'll practice each skill displayed in the **identity stress coping diagram** on the next page. In Chapters 18 and 19, you'll have the opportunity to increase self-love, self-confidence, and cultural pride by exploring the meaning and importance of your racial and cultural background to you and by increasing your confident expression of your background. Chapter 20 concludes Part Four of this workbook with skills to protect your self-love, self-confidence, and cultural pride from the negative messages you might hear or express to yourself about your racial and cultural background.

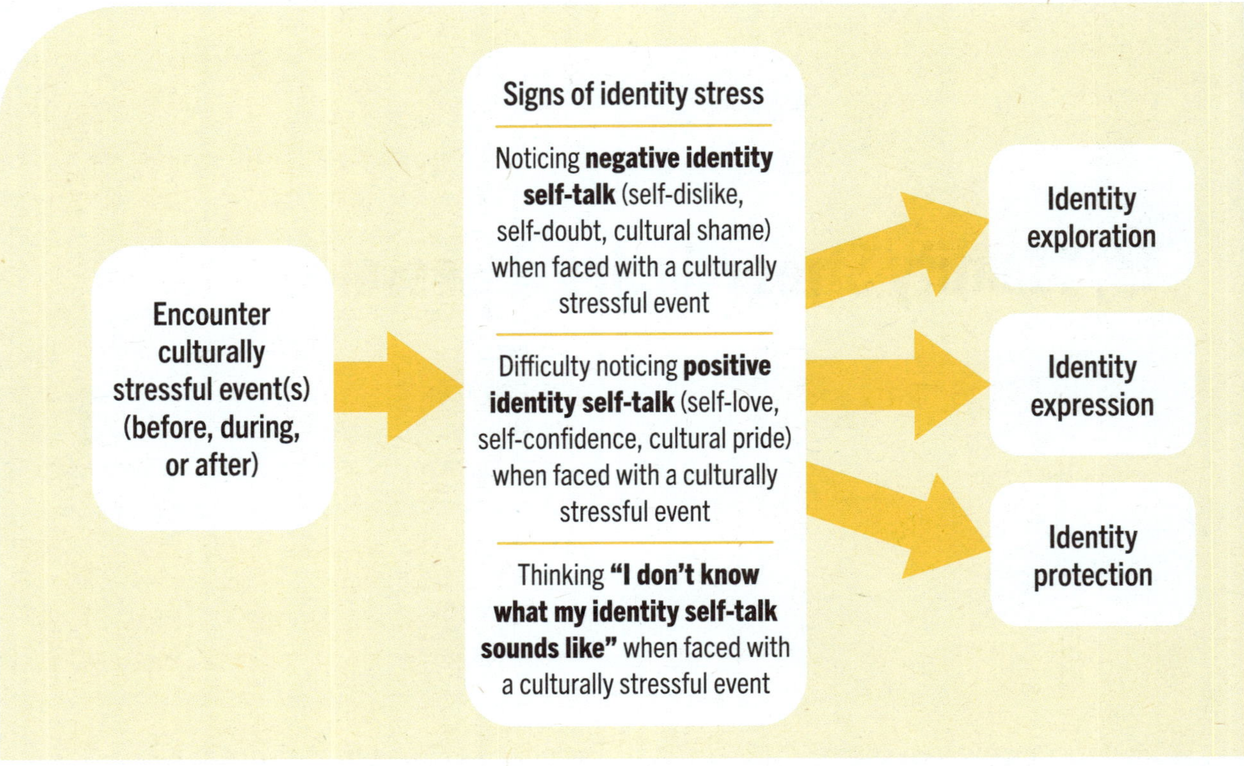

Have you used any of the coping skills in the identity stress coping diagram when faced with a culturally stressful event? Follow the steps below to explore.

1. **Identify a culturally stressful event.** Describe one past, present, or anticipated culturally stressful event that has caused you to experience identity stress. If you have any difficulty thinking of an example, look back at your responses on your My Relationship and Community Map (page 33) to help you choose one.

2. **Reflect on the identity stress coping diagram.** Review the prompts below for a quick preview of each identity stress coping decision and see if you can think of any examples of how you already practice each type of coping.

IDENTITY EXPLORATION	Before or after this culturally stressful event, have you chosen to participate in activities that have helped you *explore and clarify* the parts of your racial and cultural background that are most important to you?	○ Yes ○ No ○ Not sure
IDENTITY EXPRESSION	Before or after this culturally stressful event, have you *shared or expressed* any parts of your racial and cultural background in ways that boosted your self-love, self-confidence, or cultural pride?	○ Yes ○ No ○ Not sure

IDENTITY PROTECTION	Did you use any skills to *protect* yourself from being significantly impacted by any negative social messages you experienced from the culturally stressful event?	○ Yes ○ No ○ Not sure
Are there any additional ways that you try to cope with emotional stress that you have not already described?		○ Yes ○ No ○ Not sure

3. **Assess the result of your efforts.** How did you handle the identity stress from this culturally stressful event?

Were you pleased with how you coped with any identity stress you experienced?	○ Yes ○ No ○ Somewhat
Why or why not?	

Chapter 17: Recap and Reflect

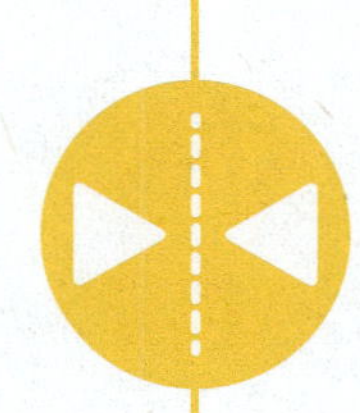

RECAP

- You need a two-pronged approach to coping with identity stress: coping skills for both building and protecting your self-love, self-confidence, and cultural pride.
- **Identity exploration** and **identity expression** are two approaches for building self-love, self-confidence, and cultural pride before facing culturally stressful events.
- **Identity protection** describes any coping skills you have for protecting your self-love, self-confidence, and cultural pride after experiencing culturally stressful events.

REFLECT

Use the questionnaire on the next page to help you determine which of the remaining chapters in Part Four you are most interested in reviewing.

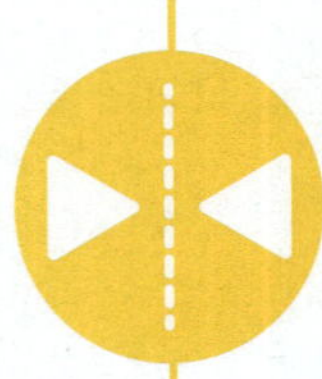

IMPACT FROM IDENTITY STRESS	RESPONSES	CHAPTER IN PART FOUR
Are there any parts of your racial and cultural background that you have yet to fully explore or have yet to determine how important this part of yourself is to you?	o Yes o No	**If yes, go to Chapter 18 (Identity Exploration)**
Are there any parts of your racial and cultural background that you are unsure how or when to express confidently?	o Yes o No	**If yes, go to Chapter 19 (Identity Expression)**
Have you ever struggled to protect yourself from the negative and critical messages you are exposed to about your racial and cultural background?	o Yes o No	**If yes, go to Chapter 20 (Identity Protection)**

18 How Can I Grow My Self-Love and Appreciation with Identity Exploration?

Whether it be conversations, traditions, stories told, media viewed, or experiences witnessed, exposure to the world around you shapes your thoughts and feelings toward your racial and cultural background. Often, it can feel most natural to go with the flow and try to fit into the norms and expectations of family, friends, and the broader society. However, sometimes you may need to carefully consider exactly what personally connects you to your racial and cultural background. You know, questions like: What parts of your background feel most important to express? How does a particular part of your background fit into the wider picture that is your overall identity? Which parts of your background might you struggle most to feel connected to?

Identity exploration describes any intentional and mindful efforts you make to clarify the personal meaning and significance of your racial and cultural background within your overall sense of self. In this chapter, you'll learn to use this coping skill to boost your self-love, self-confidence, and cultural pride.

HOW TO PRACTICE IDENTITY EXPLORATION

Here are the steps to learning identity exploration.

1. **Clarify what you hope to discover with identity exploration.** When practicing identity exploration, it can be helpful to think about the types of positive identity self-talk you're hoping to inspire with your exploration efforts. Your self-discovery goals could include learning (or being reminded of):

    - What you love about your racial and cultural background
    - Which parts of your background you want to share or express around others
    - Which parts of your background cause you to feel pride

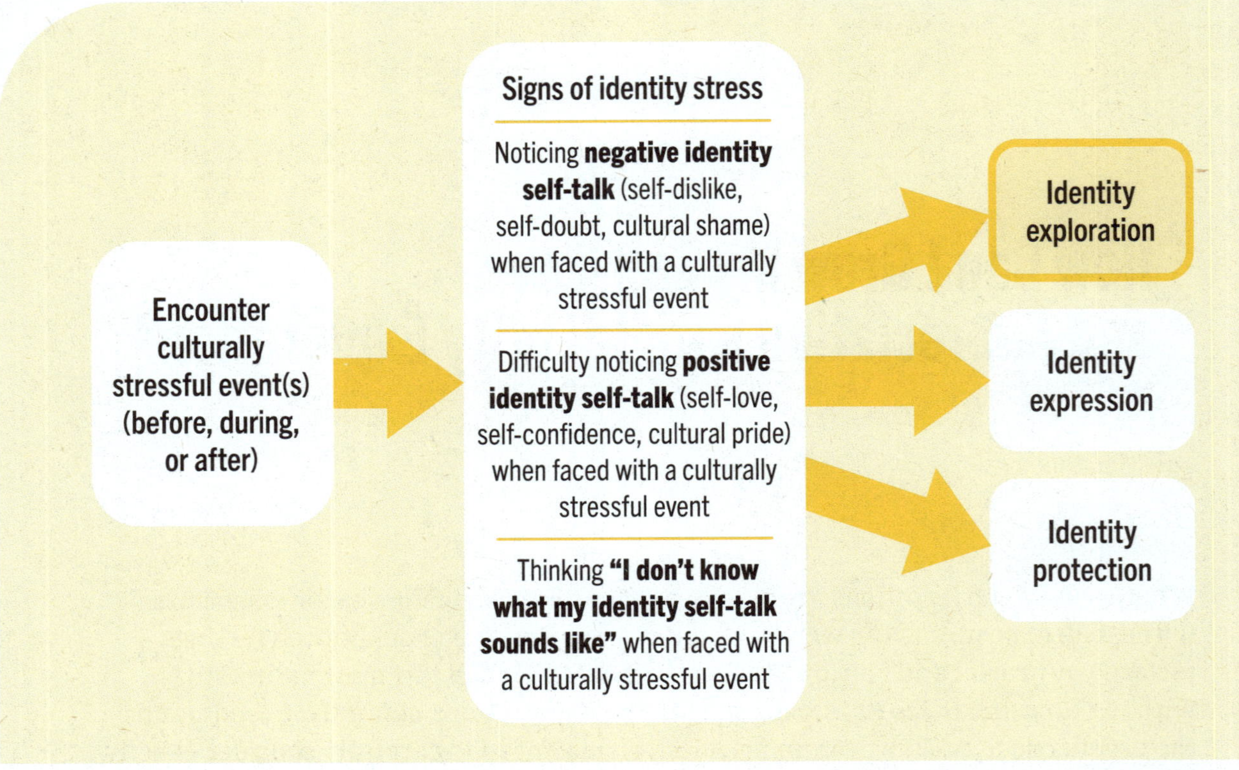

2. **Brainstorm identity exploration efforts.** The **Identity Exploration Activities list** on page 217 summarizes different ways to obtain new information about your racial and cultural background. Use this list as a tool to jump-start your brainstorming about ways to pursue your goals for growing self-love, self-confidence, or cultural pride.

3. **Create an identity exploration plan.** After brainstorming, you must actually invest time and energy into the activities you've chosen. Here (page 219) you will choose which identity exploration efforts you are most interested in making at this time and then put a plan together for when to practice identity exploration.

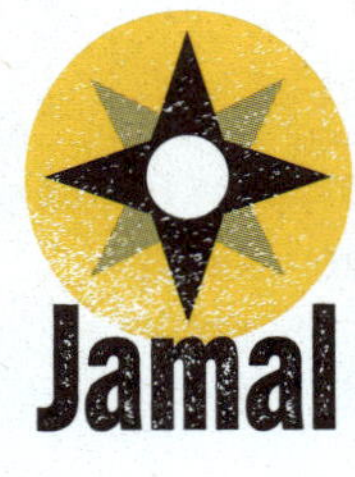

Jamal's Plan for Engaging in Identity Exploration

Jamal recently transitioned from student life to professional life. He is most familiar with the social messages he has received about being a Black male in predominantly White academic spaces and has developed an awareness of who he is and how he wants to express himself within these spaces. Now, in his new work life, he wants to explore what it means to be a Black professional. He uses the steps in this chapter to help him clarify which parts of his racial and cultural background he wants to

Identity Exploration Activities

ACTIVITIES TO COMPLETE ON YOUR OWN	ACTIVITIES TO COMPLETE WITH FAMILY AND FRIENDS	ACTIVITIES TO COMPLETE IN THE COMMUNITY
Read books about important historical events within your community	Pay close attention when older family members are telling stories related to your background	Join groups that celebrate cultural events and discuss topics related to your community
Watch TV shows/movies that feature characters from your background	Interview a family member or friend about the parts of their community they feel most connected to	Attend cultural festivals and events connected with your racial and cultural background
Take educational courses about the history of your background	Interview a family member about historical events	Experiment with sharing interests and using abilities in your Who Am I? diagram in new social spaces
Try new activities that people in your racial and cultural community are doing	Talk with friends and learn what helps them feel connected to their racial and cultural background	Travel to historic landmarks that are related to your racial and cultural background
Research details about your racial and cultural background online	Talk with family and friends about their Who Am I? diagram	Volunteer within your racial and cultural community
Read fiction that features characters from your background	Complete this workbook with family and friends	Find role models from your community and identify which of their characteristics you admire most
Follow news or social media accounts that report on current events within your community	Read books about your racial and cultural background with friends and family	Join a book club that features authors from your background
Learn cultural traditions (native language, cooking cultural foods, dances)	Watch TV shows or movies about your racial and cultural background with friends and family	Find a mentor from your community and regularly meet with them
Watch documentaries that discuss topics related to your background	Team up with your family members to trace your family lineage	Attend religious services and observances
Take time to reflect on how your goals and dreams are impacted by racial and cultural background	Talk with friends and family about what inspires their self-love, self-confidence, and cultural pride	Go to museums that showcase aspects of your background
Can you think of any other ways you can explore the important parts of your racial and cultural background? ○ Yes ○ No ○ Unsure	Describe other identity exploration activities below:	

highlight at work. He also wants to discover any new skills, values, or interests that he wants to express in this setting. Finally, he hopes his identity exploration will help him discover how to experience positive identity self-talk while in his professional setting.

1. Clarify what you hope to discover with identity exploration. Check out Jamal's goals.

WHAT I WANT TO DISCOVER	JAMAL'S RESPONSES	JAMAL'S REASONS
What I love about myself Do you hope to discover (or be reminded of) the parts of your racial and cultural background you love, appreciate, or feel most connected to?	● Yes ○ No ○ Somewhat	I want to learn how to love being my wonderful Black self in this space.
Personal abilities I can confidently use Do you hope to discover (or be reminded of) the parts of your racial and cultural background you can (or want) to express or share with others?	● Yes ○ No ○ Somewhat	I want to learn more about how my personal strengths can translate to this new workspace.
Which parts of my background bring me pride Do you hope to discover (or be reminded of) what makes you feel thankful and appreciative to be a member of your racial and cultural background or to be connected to other members within your community?	○ Yes ○ No ● Somewhat	I want to learn about and get connected with successful Black people within my field.

2. Brainstorm identity exploration efforts. After looking over the options in the Identity Exploration Activity list, Jamal felt the options below seemed the most interesting, and he was curious to see if he could use these activities to help him pursue his self-discovery goals from step 1.

POSSIBLE IDENTITY EXPLORATION EFFORT 1	**I could explore my racial and cultural background by:** experimenting with sharing interests and using abilities in my Who Am I? diagram in new social spaces. I want to see if my critical-thinking and team-building skills can help me experience positive identity self-talk like they did when I used them in college.
POSSIBLE IDENTITY EXPLORATION EFFORT 2	**I could explore my racial and cultural background by:** finding a role model and mentor at my job. There's this Black senior-level manager at my company that I could ask to meet with. It would be nice to get connected with someone who can remind me that "people like me can do this work!"
POSSIBLE IDENTITY EXPLORATION EFFORT 3	**I could explore my racial and cultural background by:** watching documentaries about successful Black professionals who achieve great things within their industries.

3. Create an identity exploration plan. As you can see from Jamal's Identity Exploration Plan below, Jamal chose to focus on two of the three options he brainstormed in step 2—expressing some of his strengths at work and finding a role model. Of note, he identified two identity exploration efforts he could use to help him find a role model—emailing the senior-level manager to request a meeting and drafting a list of questions to help him get the most out of their meeting. He realizes that these efforts alone are unlikely to be enough to accomplish his self-discovery goals. But he plans to revisit the three steps in this chapter regularly to keep a clear and focused eye on how he is building positive self-talk in this new setting.

	CHOOSE YOUR EXPLORATION EFFORTS	WHEN DO YOU WANT TO PRACTICE?
IDENTITY EXPLORATION EFFORT 1	Signing up to take lead on a team project	I want to try to do this within the first two months of being in this position. I think challenging myself to do this early will help me learn how to use my critical-thinking and team-building skills at this job.
IDENTITY EXPLORATION EFFORT 2	Contacting the Black senior-level mentor to schedule a follow-up meeting	The last time I saw my mentor, they told me to reach out anytime. I want to send them an email by this Friday to hopefully meet sometime in the next couple of weeks.
IDENTITY EXPLORATION EFFORT 3	Creating a list of questions to ask my senior-level mentor about how they achieved their career goals within the company	I keep a mental note of how my mentor carries themselves in meetings and around our coworkers. I just have a few questions about how they keep such a calm yet strong presence despite our coworkers being so insensitive sometimes.

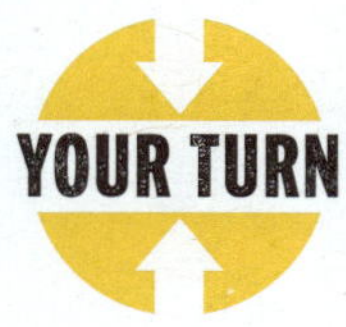

1. Clarify what you hope to discover with identity exploration. Use the **My Self-Discovery Goals worksheet** (page 222) to help you identify any self-discovery goals that you have. Also, feel free to add any goals that do not fall within these three goal categories.

My Self-Discovery Goals

WHAT I WANT TO DISCOVER	YOUR RESPONSES	YOUR REASONS
What I love about myself Do you hope to discover (or be reminded of) the parts of your racial and cultural background you love, appreciate, or feel most connected to?	○ Yes ○ No ○ Somewhat	
Personal abilities I can confidently use Do you hope to discover (or be reminded of) the parts of your racial and cultural background you can (or want) to express or share with others?	○ Yes ○ No ○ Somewhat	
Which parts of my background bring me pride Do you hope to discover (or be reminded of) what makes you feel thankful and appreciative to be a member of your racial and cultural background or to be connected to other members within your community?	○ Yes ○ No ○ Somewhat	
Can you think of any other self-discovery goals besides what you listed above?	○ Yes ○ No ○ Somewhat	Describe additional goals:

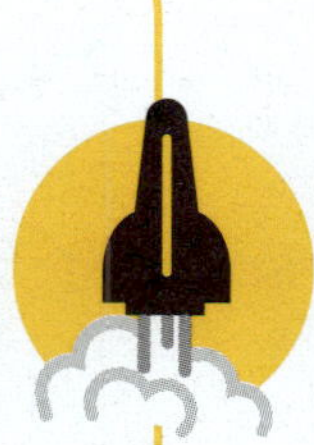

Power Up! Tips for Boosting Your Empowered Coping

- **Creating self-discovery goals can be hard.** If you are having difficulty thinking of self-discovery goals for step 1, consider looking back at the Who Am I? diagram you filled in on page 14. Then use these questions to help you come up with your goals.
  - Discovering your "I am": When filling in your Who Am I? diagram, was there any part of your racial and cultural background that you were unsure how to represent on your diagram? If so, a self-discovery goal could be obtaining more information about the unknown parts of your background.
  - Discovering your "I like": When filling in your Who Am I? diagram, did you have any difficulty thinking of interests that were connected with (or inspired by) your racial and cultural background? If so, a self-discovery goal could be learning about traditional activities within your community and exploring whether participating in these activities inspires pride.
  - Discovering your "I can do": When filling in your Who Am I? diagram, did you struggle to connect any of your strengths with your racial and cultural background? If so, a self-discovery goal could be learning to use your strengths in a way that helps you feel connected to your background.
  - Discovering your "I care about": When filling in your Who Am I? diagram, did you struggle to see how your racial and cultural background informed your values? If so, a self-discovery goal could be learning what many people in your community value and discovering if any of these values can help you feel more connected to your community.
- **Calling in your workbook navigators:** Consider talking to your workbook navigators to help you come up with some ideas of activities that might help you discover what you might love and appreciate about your background.
- **Use the Recap and Reflect.** Before putting your plan into action, take a quick look at the reflection prompts in the Recap and Reflect at the end of this chapter. Try to keep these questions in mind so that you can use your identity exploration efforts to gather information to answer each prompt. Importantly, this will help assure you progress toward reaching your self-discovery goals!

2. Brainstorm identity exploration efforts. In the table below, describe at least three identity exploration efforts you would be willing to use to pursue your self-discovery goals at this time. Remember to use the Identity Exploration Activities list on page 219.

My Identity Exploration Efforts

POSSIBLE IDENTITY EXPLORATION EFFORT 1	
POSSIBLE IDENTITY EXPLORATION EFFORT 2	
POSSIBLE IDENTITY EXPLORATION EFFORT 3	

3. Create an identity exploration plan. Now use the worksheet below to help you prioritize which identity exploration efforts you are most interested in making at this time and then put a plan together for when you want to practice identity exploration.

My Identity Exploration Plan

	CHOOSE YOUR EXPLORATION EFFORTS	WHEN DO YOU WANT TO PRACTICE?
IDENTITY EXPLORATION EFFORT 1		
IDENTITY EXPLORATION EFFORT 2		
IDENTITY EXPLORATION EFFORT 3		

Chapter 18: Recap and Reflect

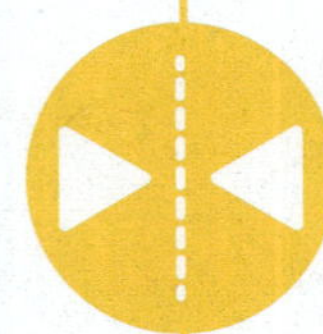

RECAP

- **Identity exploration** is any intentional and mindful efforts you make to clarify the personal meaning and significance of your racial and cultural background within your overall sense of self.
- The steps for practicing the identity exploration skill include:
    1. Clarify what you hope to discover with identity exploration.
    2. Brainstorm identity exploration efforts.
    3. Create an identity exploration plan.

REFLECT

Hopefully, you have had an opportunity to practice using your identity exploration plan. Before moving forward, take a moment to think about what you learned about identity exploration and how you hope to use this skill to cope with identity stress moving forward. To do so, answer the questions below.

Calling in your workbook navigators: You may also find it helpful to review your answers to these questions with your workbook navigators, as they can share ways their identity exploration efforts helped them along their journey of self-discovery.

Did you learn or see anything *new or unsuspected* about your racial and cultural background from your identity exploration? If so, what was your reaction to this information about your background?

Did you learn or see anything *inspiring* or that *made you feel proud* to be a member of your racial and cultural background from your identity exploration? If so, what did you discover?

Did you learn or see anything you *disagreed* with or that made you *feel uncomfortable* from your identity exploration? If so, what did you discover?

Did you discover anything important about your Who Am I? diagram, such as any new *abilities, interests,* or *values* you want to prioritize in your daily life?

Did you discover anything from your identity exploration that has helped you to grow your self-love, self-confidence, or cultural pride?

19 How Can I Grow My Self-Love and Appreciation with Identity Expression?

As we discover the parts of our racial and cultural background that we feel most connected to, we can continue growing our self-love, self-confidence, and cultural pride by practicing **identity expression.** This coping skill is all about finding as many relationships and community spaces in our lives as we can to authentically express various aspects of our racial and cultural background. It would be great if we lived in a world where POCs could be carefree in how they choose to express and showcase their backgrounds to the world around them. But, as you've been learning, culturally stressful events can expose POCs to negative and critical social messages that can complicate knowing when, where, and how to confidently express who they are.

In this chapter, you'll learn to use this coping tool to help you identify the safest spaces where you want to practice identity expression and learn how to create an identity expression plan that builds your tolerance for any discomfort caused by expressing yourself. Let's get started by first seeing how one of our navigators practiced identity expression when she experienced identity stress. Then you will have a chance at the end of the chapter to start practicing yourself.

HOW TO PRACTICE IDENTITY EXPRESSION

Here are the steps to learning identity expression.

1. **Clarify the focus of your identity expression efforts.** Identity expression efforts include any behaviors, interests, or activities related to your background that you choose to express or share within your relationships and community

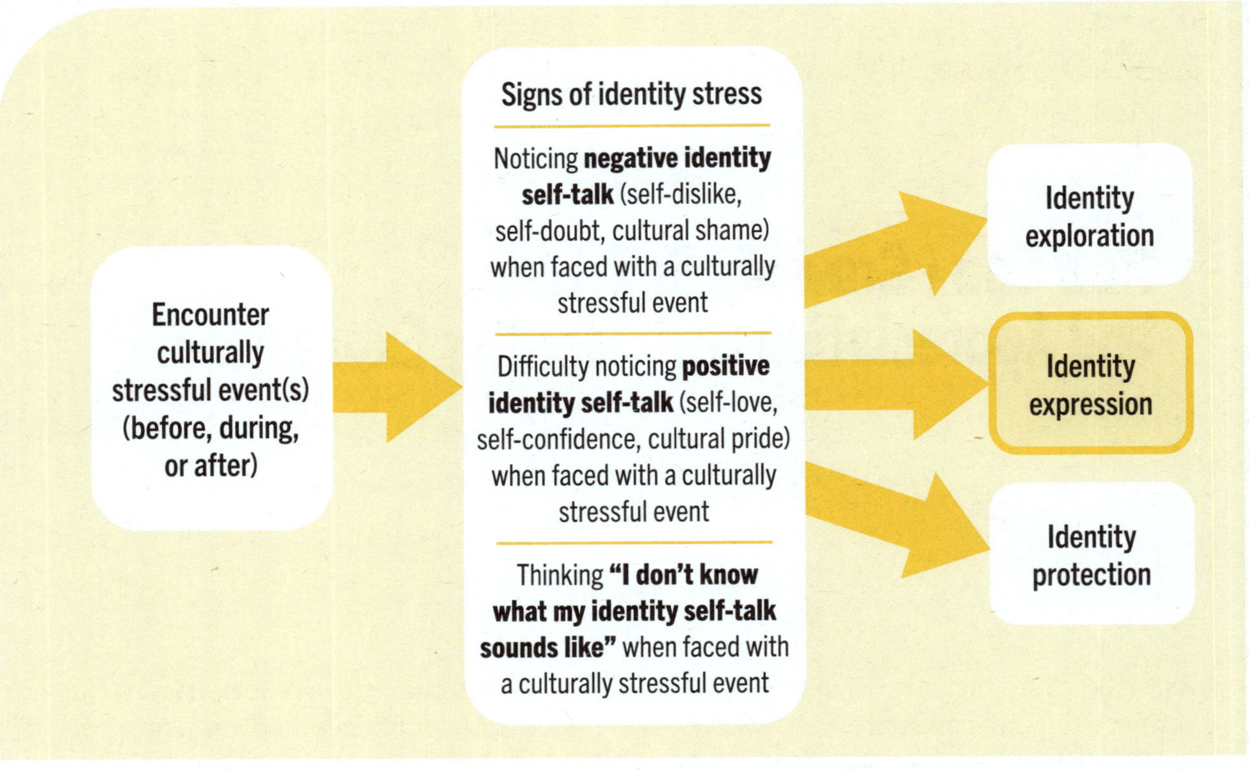

spaces. For some, such self-expression inspires feelings of power, hope, and belongingness. You know, feeling able to be your true self can be a liberating and exciting feeling! Of course, you may not always feel you can share or express yourself with freedom and originality. But for now, check out the Identity Expression Examples table on the facing page, which includes some ways POCs may choose to confidently be themselves. This is not a complete list, but hopefully it will give you some ideas of what identity expression efforts you can make.

Pause and Reflect on Your Identity Expression

Look back at your latest Who Am I? diagram (Chapter 1) to familiarize yourself with the interests, strengths, and values that are most connected to your racial and cultural background. Then *circle or check off* examples in the Identity Expression Examples table that would help you share and express your Who Am I? diagram.

IDENTITY EXPRESSION EXAMPLES

- ☐ Wear a specific hairstyle (natural hair, colorful weave or braids)
- ☐ Eat cultural foods in public (cafeteria or work)
- ☐ Wear cultural/traditional clothing
- ☐ Share interests that are related to your racial and cultural background (music, TV, art, food)
- ☐ Date who you want to date (publicly or privately)
- ☐ Share stories about your racial and cultural background
- ☐ Use slang terms or phrases often expressed within your racial and cultural community
- ☐ Maintain an observance of cultural traditions, such as religious prayers
- ☐ Choose to pursue academic/career goals that honor your racial and cultural community
- ☐ Learn to and openly speak your native language
- ☐ Choose *not* to engage in certain behaviors because doing so does not fit within your cultural beliefs
- ☐ Celebrate cultural holidays
- ☐ Inform others about current events impacting your racial and cultural community
- ☐ Attend religious ceremonies/services
- ☐ Create arts and crafts that celebrate racial and cultural experiences
- ☐ Stay up to date on current events impacting your racial and cultural community
- ☐ Participate in activities or projects that improve your racial and cultural community
- ☐ Invite people not within your racial and cultural community to participate in cultural celebrations/traditions
- ☐ Support and celebrate the work of other members within your racial and cultural community
- ☐ Protect time to connect with family
- ☐ Attend cultural festivals/celebrations
- ☐ Read books that focus on your racial and cultural background
- ☐ Speak up against injustices/address the issues that impact your community
- ☐ Engage in and teach others about cultural traditions (dance, cooking, storytelling)
- ☐ Listen to and share your cultural music with others
- ☐ Ask people to pronounce your name correctly
- ☐ Publicly observe your faith
- ☐ **List any other identity expression ideas you can think of:**

2. Consider the costs of identity expression. It would be great if identity expression were this simple—select how you want to express yourself and then just do it anywhere and everywhere. Unfortunately, identity expression can come at a cost. This can include the social, emotional, resource, and safety costs of trying to authentically express your racial and cultural background in social spaces that do not feel supportive or safe. It can be important to identify any costs that you anticipate, as doing so will help you create a safer plan for identity expression.

3. Brainstorm ways to support your identity expression efforts. Identity expression is not an all-or-nothing experience. In this chapter, you will learn about the following types of identity expression:

- **Open expression.** These are moments when you may feel empowered to openly and freely express your background—like wearing your natural hair down or openly speaking in your cultural language.
- **Selective expression.** These are moments when you may have learned that changing how you speak, dress, or carry yourself within a certain social space will help minimize any social, resource, safety, or emotional costs you anticipate. This type of expression is often referred to as "code switching."
- **Undiscovered expression.** This type of expression happens whenever you run into new people or enter new places without knowing how safe it is to authentically express yourself. In these moments, you are tasked with choosing how you want to express yourself until you get more information about whether you will feel safe and supported to express yourself more openly.

4. Create an identity expression plan. Now it's time to put a plan together for how and when you want to practice identity expression. Remember, this coping skill is all about finding as many spaces as you can to express your racial and cultural background in ways that hopefully boost your self-love, self-confidence, and cultural pride. And, because identity expression can, at times, be costly (step 2), it is important to have an identity expression plan that considers when, where, and with whom you want to express your racial and cultural background.

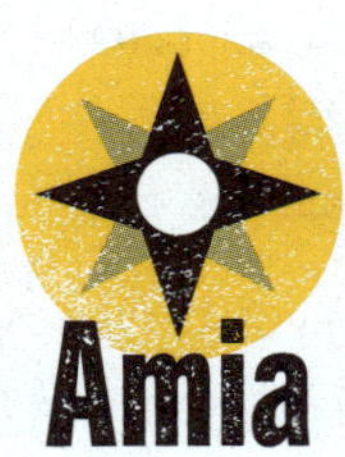

Amia's Plan for Engaging in Identity Expression

Since immigrating to the United States with her family, Amia has been teased and criticized for her religion. The target of others' insensitive comments has also been Amia's choice to wear hijab—a religious and cultural observance that she never thought twice about before moving to the United States. She recently met a Muslim female classmate who has chosen not to wear hijab at their school, which then made Amia question her own observance. Often Amia wakes up dreading the consequences of wearing hijab at school. Sometimes she thinks, "If I keep wearing hijab at my school, everyone will continue to stare at me and make me feel uncomfortable." Amia decided she wanted to use the steps in this chapter to help her regain confidence in wearing hijab because doing so boosts her cultural pride by making her feel closer to God and her community.

1. Clarify the focus of your identity expression efforts. After reviewing the Identity Expressions Examples on page 229, Amia chose to pursue the following identity expression goals as a way of rebuilding and strengthening her positive identity self-talk related to her background.

IDENTITY EXPRESSION GOAL 1	**I want to express and share my racial and cultural background by:** observing my faith. I really want to keep up with my daily prayers and attending religious ceremonies/events.
IDENTITY EXPRESSION GOAL 2	**I want to express and share my racial and cultural background by:** wearing cultural/traditional clothing. I want to keep wearing my hijab. That's really important to me.
IDENTITY EXPRESSION GOAL 3	**I want to express and share my racial and cultural background by:** staying up to date on and discussing current events impacting my racial and cultural community. I want to stay knowledgeable about what's happening in my home country.

2. Consider the cost of identity expression. As we can see from Amia's responses below, identity expression is not without cost or consequence. Importantly, Amia's responses show that her past experiences with culturally stressful events as well as what she observes elsewhere in the world can raise concern about identity expression. Please note that step 2 here is not intended to convince you to avoid expressing yourself. Instead, my hope is that it will give you important information that you can use in step 3 to help you select the people and places who seem most and least likely to cause these concerns to become a reality.

TYPES OF COSTS	AMIA'S EXAMPLES
Social costs Do you anticipate that your self-expression will be met with rejection, criticism, or judgment?	I worry that wearing hijab will cause my classmates to keep teasing me and they will not want to be friends with me because of some of the mean things people say about Muslims.
Resource costs Do you anticipate that your self-expression will lead to a removal or denial of needed or wanted resources?	I am not sure about this right now. But sometimes I wonder if my teachers are less willing to help me because of my Muslim background.
Safety costs Do you anticipate that your self-expression will be met with threatened or experienced physical harm?	I worry that wearing hijab in parts of my city could lead to physical harm—especially during times when the local news broadcasts stories about any terrorist attacks happening in the world.
Emotional costs Do you anticipate that your self-expression will cause overwhelming bodily and emotional discomfort?	If I continue to wear hijab at this school, I'll likely feel so anxious and uncomfortable that I'll just be thinking about leaving school all class.

3. Brainstorm ways to support your identity expression efforts. Balancing open and selective expression can be an all too familiar and required dance for many POCs. This is a reality that Amia is becoming more and more aware of as she continues to adjust to life in the United States. In the worksheet below, Amia was able to identify several people and places where she feels able to let her guard down and freely express her faith. Also, she used step 3 to remind herself to be cautious about how freely she expresses these parts of her identity around certain people and in certain places that have proven to be culturally stressful in the past.

TYPES OF EXPRESSION	MY RESPONSES
Open expression *In which relationships **am I able to openly and freely** practice identity expression?*	I feel able to openly express myself in these **relationships:** my mom, middle sister, cousin, friends at mosque, ESL teacher, and my two POC classmates and youth leader
Open expression *In which community spaces **am I able to openly and freely** practice identity expression?*	I feel able to openly express myself in these **community spaces:** my cousin's house, mosque, home
Selective expression *In which relationships do I feel as if I **must consider limiting how openly and freely** I practice identity expression?*	I feel like I will consider limiting how openly I express myself in these **relationships:** White classmates, history teacher
Selective expression *In which community spaces do I feel as if I **must consider limiting how openly and freely** I practice identity expression?*	I feel like I will consider limiting how openly I express myself in these **community spaces:** School or public transportation
Undiscovered expression *In which relationships have you **yet to discover how comfortable you are** with openly and freely practicing identity expression?*	I have yet to discover how I want to express myself in these **relationships:** when around many of my POC classmates, several school administrators, and teachers
Undiscovered expression *In which community spaces have you **yet to discover how comfortable you are** with openly and freely practicing identity expression?*	I have yet to discover how I want to express myself in these **community spaces:** my local mall, when spending time in cities/towns surrounding where I live

4. Create an identity expression plan. While Amia still feels threatened by ongoing culturally stressful events within her school, she feels proud that she was able to use this chapter to find options to boost her positive identity self-talk. See how she used this identity expression plan worksheet to help her plan for open, selective, and undiscovered expression of each identity expression goal.

IDENTITY EXPRESSION GOALS	OPEN EXPRESSION	SELECTIVE EXPRESSION	UNDISCOVERED EXPRESSION
Wearing hijab	Wearing hijab with different vibrant colors: I actually really like being fashionable and mixing it up	Wearing hijab, but wearing only neutral colors so I don't bring too much attention to myself	Wearing neutral-colored hijabs until I learn more about the people I am with and their beliefs about my culture
Daily prayers	Praying openly and asking my Muslim friends to pray alongside me	Finding private places to pray where people won't really see me	Praying privately and not discussing my daily prayers until I learn more about the people around me and their beliefs about my culture
Attending religious services	Making sure to attend weekly events at my Islamic Community Center	Not talking openly about the religious events I attend at my mosque	Not talking openly about what we do at the Islamic Community Center until I learn more about the people around me and their beliefs about my culture

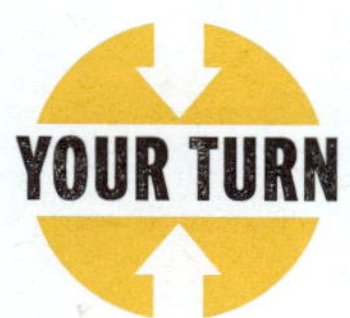

Use the following steps to help you find the identity expression efforts that you can use to grow and maintain your self-love, self-confidence, and cultural pride.

1. **Clarify the focus of your identity expression goals.** In the worksheet on the next page, describe three ways you want to prioritize identity expression at this time. Remember to use the Identity Expression Examples (page 229) and your workbook navigators to help you come up with some ideas.

My Identity Expression Goals

IDENTITY EXPRESSION GOAL 1	**I want to express and share my racial and cultural background by:**
IDENTITY EXPRESSION GOAL 2	**I want to express and share my racial and cultural background by:**
IDENTITY EXPRESSION GOAL 3	**I want to express and share my racial and cultural background by:**

2. **Consider the costs of identity expression.** In the worksheet on the facing page, describe any costs that may influence when, where, or how you decide to engage in your identity expression efforts.

Costs That Might Influence My Identity Expression Efforts

TYPES OF COSTS	MY RESPONSES
Social costs Do you anticipate that your self-expression will be met with rejection, criticism, or judgment?	
Resource costs Do you anticipate that your self-expression will lead to a removal or denial of needed or wanted resources?	
Safety costs Do you anticipate that your self-expression will be met with threatened or experienced physical harm?	
Emotional costs Do you anticipate that your self-expression will cause overwhelming bodily and emotional discomfort?	
Other costs Describe any other costs you are concerned about experiencing:	

3. **Brainstorm ways to support your identity expression efforts.** Use the worksheet below to reflect on the different levels of support and safety offered by the people and places around you. Feel free to look back at your My Relationship and Community Map in Chapter 2 to help you complete Step 3.

Where I Can Practice Identity Expression

TYPES OF EXPRESSION	YOUR RESPONSES
Open expression *In which relationships **am I able to openly and freely** practice identity expression?*	I feel able to openly express myself in these **relationships:**
Open expression *In which community spaces **am I able to openly and freely** practice identity expression?*	I feel able to openly express myself in these **community spaces:**
Selective expression *In which relationships do I feel as if I **must consider limiting how openly and freely** I practice identity expression?*	I feel like I will consider limiting how openly I express myself in these **relationships:**
Selective expression *In which community spaces do I feel as if I **must consider limiting how openly and freely** I practice identity expression?*	I feel like I will consider limiting how openly I express myself in these **community spaces:**
Undiscovered expression *In which relationships have you **yet to discover how comfortable you are** with openly and freely practicing identity expression?*	I have yet to discover how I want to express myself in these **relationships:**
Undiscovered expression *In which community spaces have you **yet to discover how comfortable you are** with openly and freely practicing identity expression?*	I have yet to discover how I want to express myself in these **community spaces:**

4. Create an identity expression plan. Now it's time to put a plan together for how and when you want to practice identity expression. Use the instructions and worksheet below to help you clarify how you will try to express yourself within your surroundings.

My Identity Expression Plan

1. **List identity expression goals.** First, list examples of identity expression efforts you can make.
2. **Define open expression.** Under "open expression," describe what openly expressing your racial and cultural background looks like in the social spaces where you feel the most safe and supported to do so.
3. **Define selective expression.** Under "selective expression," describe what selectively expressing your racial and cultural background looks like in social spaces where you are most concerned about experiencing social, resource, safety, or emotional costs.
4. **Define undiscovered expression.** Finally, under "undiscovered expression," describe how you might go about discovering how you can express your racial and cultural background in social spaces you remain unsure about.

IDENTITY EXPRESSION GOALS	OPEN EXPRESSION	SELECTIVE EXPRESSION	UNDISCOVERED EXPRESSION

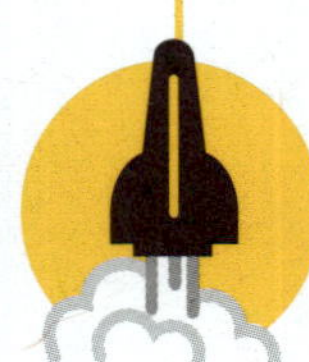

Power Up! Tips for Boosting Your Empowered Coping

To assist you in using identity expression to build your positive identity self-talk:

- **Remember to be mindful.** When you have the opportunity to engage in open expression, try to remain mindful during these moments and truly savor any self-love, self-confidence, and cultural pride you experience.
- **Keep in mind that selective expression can still be empowering.** Try to view your selective expression in a way that maintains your positive identity self-talk. Reflect on how your expression (no matter how subtle) remains a reflection of your love and appreciation toward your background.
- **Keep your self-compassion skills close.** Unfortunately, there are times when avoiding identity expression feels like the best way to minimize any unwanted costs or outcomes. When this happens, it is important to use the self-compassion skills in Chapters 5, 11, and 16 and continue taking advantage of other social spaces that offer more freedom to openly be yourself.
- **Check out the Recap and Reflect.** Before putting your plan into action, take a quick look at the reflection prompts in Recap and Reflect at the end of this chapter. Try to keep these questions in mind as you practice identity expression. Doing so will help you gather information to answer each prompt!

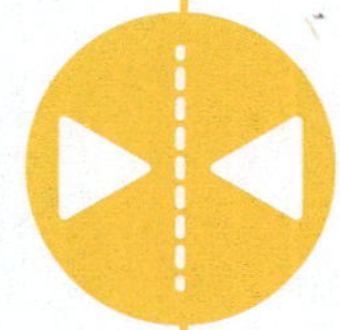

Chapter 19: Recap and Reflect

RECAP

- **Identity expression** describes any behaviors, interests, or activities that you feel are important representations of your identity that you want to express or share within your relationships and community spaces.
- The steps for practicing the identity expression skill include:
  1. Clarify the focus of your identity expression goals.
  2. Identify any costs of identity expression.
  3. Brainstorm ways to support identity expression efforts.
  4. Create an identity expression plan.

REFLECT

Hopefully, you have had an opportunity to practice using your identity expression plan. Before moving forward, take a moment to think about what you learned about identity expression and how you hope to use this skill to cope with identity stress. To do so, answer the following questions.

Calling in your workbook navigators: You may also find it helpful to review your answers to these questions with your workbook navigators, as they can share ways they've navigated the costs of identity expression and how their identity expression has contributed to their positive identity self-talk.

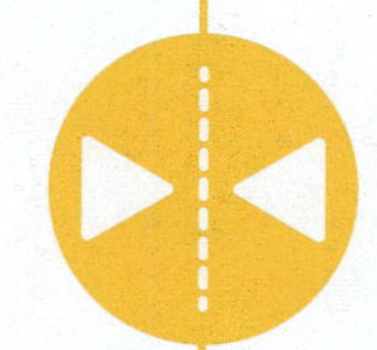

Did you learn any new approaches for helping you express yourself?

Are there any social, resource, safety, or emotional costs that you have learned how to minimize or handle so that you can more openly express your racial and cultural background? If so, please describe.

Have your identity expression efforts helped you boost your self-love, self-confidence, or cultural pride? If so, describe what types of positive identity self-talk you have been experiencing.

During your identity expression, did you learn anything new to add to your Who Am I? diagram (Chapter 1), such as any new interests, abilities, or values?

20 How Can I Protect the Self-Love and Appreciation I Am Building?

Imagine this scenario: You've decided to throw yourself a big birthday party with all of your favorite people. As your guests arrive, you notice all the love you're feeling and how much you're looking forward to an amazing night. The next thing you know, a group of uninvited guests shows up screaming "Let's party!" These particular guests were not invited for a reason. Historically they have criticized you, judged you, and talked behind your back—you know, all the things you don't want at your birthday party.

So what do you do? When I pose this question to the teens and young adults I work with, I typically hear some version of "I'm going to kick them out." For most people, such an assertive demand would work. But these uninvited guests are relentless and stubborn.

Identity exploration and expression are important to discovering and growing self-love and cultural appreciation, but you need **identity protection** to guard yourself from the uninvited "guests." In this chapter, these uninvited guests are the lingering negative identity self-talk that interferes with your self-love and cultural appreciation. And just like the unwanted party guests, this self-talk may not always be easy to eject. But you can learn skills to protect yourself from such thoughts. Your life and relationship with your racial and cultural background is a party you can enjoy and thrive in—even when uninvited guests intrude.

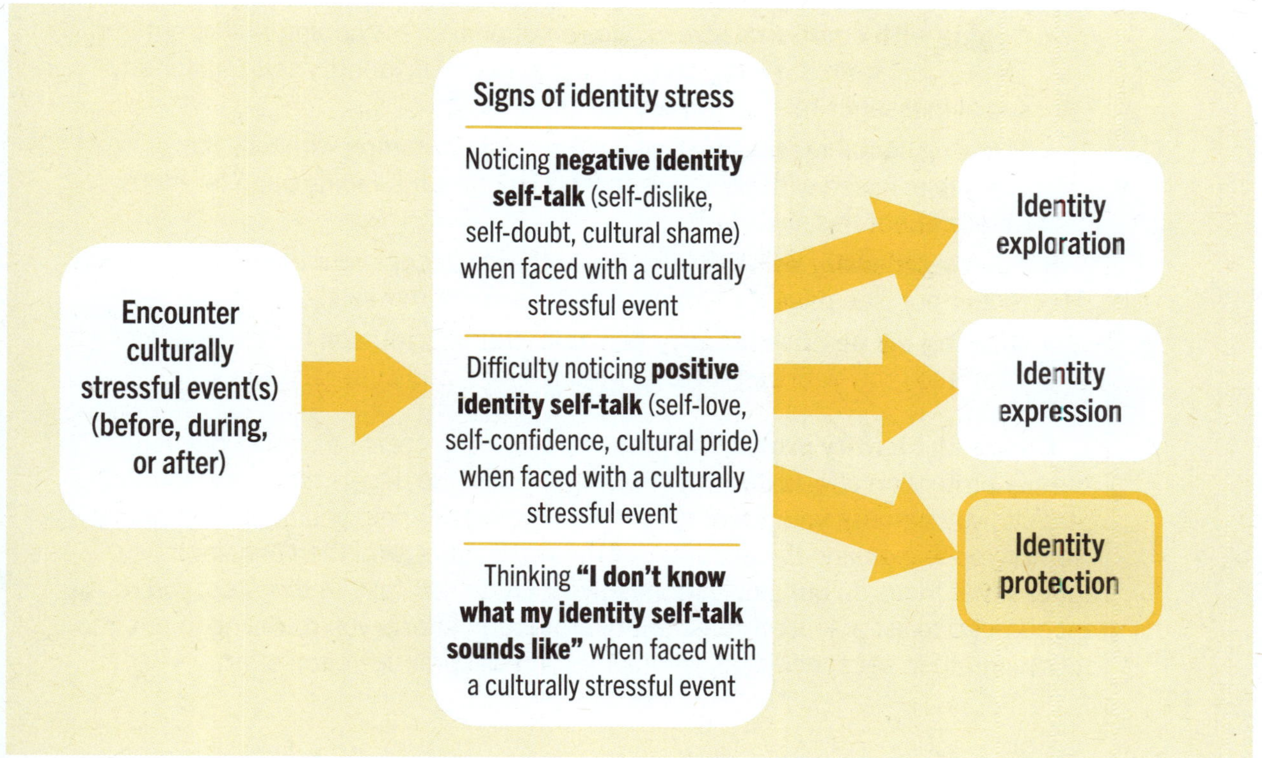

HOW TO PRACTICE IDENTITY PROTECTION

Here are the steps to learning identity protection.

1. **Notice your negative identity self-talk.** The first step of practicing identity protection is to understand how your negative identity self-talk is impacting you. Possibly your negative thoughts are complicating your positive identity self-talk or even interfering with your identity expression. Or maybe such thoughts cut a bit deeper and leave a strong emotional impact. In any case, knowing how your negative identity self-talk is impacting you can support your ability to create a more effective identity protection plan.

2. **Brainstorm options for protecting yourself.** Now it's time to brainstorm identity protection efforts that will help you limit how deep these impacts become. Step 2 is all about answering the question "What efforts can I make in this moment to protect my self-love, self-confidence, and cultural pride from this negative identity self-talk?" Remember, the goal of identity protection efforts is not to abruptly stop negative identity self-talk. Instead, these efforts focus on helping you practice the following identity protection skills.

- **Coping with emotional stress.** Use emotional stress coping skills from Part Two to heal from the emotional impact of negative identity self-talk (or any social messages related to your self-talk).
- **Filtering social messages.** Call out any misinformation within social messages linked with your identity self-talk (see the facing page for more details about this skill).
- **Filtering identity self-talk.** Know whether to accept your identity self-talk as fact or not (see page 244 for more details about this skill).
- **Growing my positive identity self-talk.** Remind yourself to keep making efforts to grow your self-love, self-confidence, and cultural pride.

3. Create an identity protection plan. Now you can create a plan to put your identity protection efforts into action. Even when some negative identity self-talk persists, you can use your identity protection efforts to help you heal emotionally, prompt you to examine the accuracy of these thoughts, and then engage in actions that focus on building your positive identity self-talk. In this step, you're encouraged to list at least three identity protection efforts you're willing to put into action and then set specific goals for when you will practice each effort.

√TIP SHEET

TIP SHEETS FOR FILTERING SOCIAL MESSAGES AND IDENTITY SELF-TALK

In the diagram below, do you notice the dotted circle in the middle? It symbolizes a filter that protects the "Me" figure in the center. You may use a filtration system to remove any health-harming substances from the water you drink. Similarly, when you notice identity stress, you need an identity filtration system to remove social messages and identity self-talk that shouldn't be accepted as absolute fact, leaving in your mind only the ones you can trust.

One way to establish an identity filter is to have a short list of questions that help you pause and carefully think through how you want to respond to the social messages you receive and the thoughts you have about your racial and cultural background. In these Tip Sheets you will see several questions for **filtering social messages** and several questions for **filtering identity self-talk.** Try them out and see if any of them help you with identity protection.

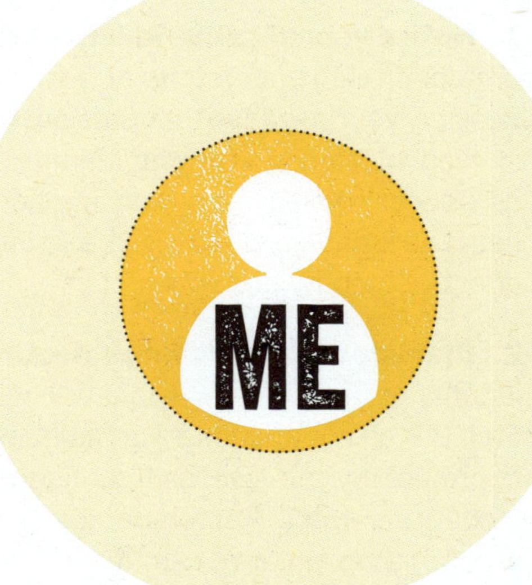

Tip Sheet: Filtering Social Messages

First, look back at the positive stereotypes you listed on page 202 and negative stereotypes on page 205 in Chapter 16, and think about which social messages are most strongly associated with your identity self-talk (positive or negative). Then, focusing on one social message at a time, use the following questions to assess how trustworthy that social message is at that particular moment. (You can repeat this exercise with any social messages that feel connected with your identity self-talk.) Also, feel free to add any filter questions that will help you make sense of the social messages around you.

Can I Trust This Social Message?

FACTUAL MESSAGE	Describe any evidence that: ☐ **Supports** this social message as an accurate representation of you or your community ☐ **Does *not* support** this social message as an accurate representation of you or your community
WHO AM I TRULY?	What parts of your Who Am I? diagram remain *true* and *unchanged* no matter what these social messages say about your racial and cultural background? ☐ "I am still . . . " ☐ "I still like to do . . . " ☐ "I can still do . . . " ☐ "I still care about . . . "
IDENTITY-CONSISTENT MESSAGE	Is there any part of this social message that is consistent with your Who Am I? diagram? ○ If so, what efforts can you make in your daily life to strengthen your belief in this social message? ○ If not, what efforts can you make to remind yourself (and possibly others) that this social message does not represent who you are?
YOUR CONCLUSION	Is there any meaningful information you can take away from your responses to the filter questions above? If so, describe any conclusion(s):

Tip Sheet: Filtering Identity Self-Talk

First, think about your identity self-talk (both positive and negative). Then, focusing on one thought at a time, use the following questions to assess how trustworthy each thought is and how you want to respond to its presence within your BEAT. (You can repeat this exercise with any other identity self-talk thoughts.) Feel free to add any filter questions that will help you make sense of the identity self-talk you hear often.

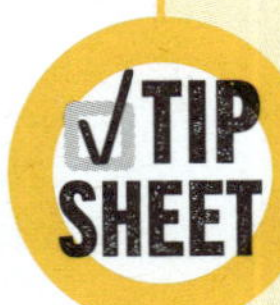

Should I Trust My Identity Self-Talk?

WHO AM I TRULY?

What parts of your Who Am I? diagram remain *true* and *unchanged* no matter what your current self-talk says?

- ☐ "I am still . . . "
- ☐ "I still like to do . . . "
- ☐ "I can still do . . . "
- ☐ "I still care about . . . "

IDENTITY-CONSISTENT THOUGHT

Is this self-talk consistent with how you want to see yourself?

- o If so, what efforts can you make in your daily life to strengthen your belief in this thought in ways that are helpful to you?
- o If not, what efforts can you make to help you to have more self-loving, self-confidence, and cultural pride thoughts?

SUPPORTIVE THOUGHT

Is this self-talk guiding you closer to your goals (the things in life you want to achieve) or values (what you care most about)?

- o If so, then how can you use this thought to help you achieve your goals and live according to your values?
- o If not, then what efforts can you make moving forward to strengthen your self-loving, self-confident, and cultural pride thoughts in ways that help you achieve your goals and live according to your values?

YOUR CONCLUSION

Is there any meaningful information you can take away from your responses to the filter questions above? If so, describe any conclusion(s):

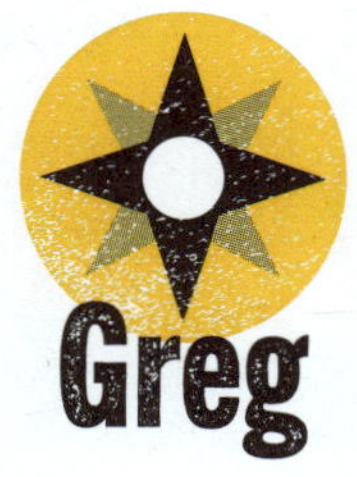

Greg's Plan for Engaging in Identity Protection

Greg has gotten stuck in thoughts like "I am acting too White" after his close friends teased him about his musical interests and academic motivations. See how he used the steps below to help him brainstorm options for protecting his self-love, self-confidence, and cultural pride from this lingering thought.

1. Notice your negative identity self-talk. Greg's answers indicate that his negative identity self-talk is interfering mostly with his ability to experience self-love and cultural pride. Although negative identity self-talk can trigger strong emotional responses or reduce self-confidence, Greg did not notice his self-talk impacting him in these ways.

THINGS TO THINK ABOUT	MY RESPONSES
What negative identity self-talk are you focusing on?	"I am acting too White."
Is this self-talk causing you any **emotional stress** in this moment?	○ Yes ● No ○ Somewhat
Explain your answer:	I am okay right now. Not feeling too upset.
Is this self-talk impacting your **self-love** in this moment?	● Yes ○ No ○ Somewhat
Explain your answer:	I keep questioning if my music interests are too White.
Is this self-talk impacting your **self-confidence** in this moment?	○ Yes ○ No ● Somewhat
Explain your answer:	I like what I like, but I sometimes doubt if it's okay to share my interests with people.
Is this self-talk impacting your **cultural pride** in this moment?	● Yes ○ No ○ Somewhat
Explain your answer:	Sometimes I just feel so different from my Latino friends. I hate to say it, but sometimes they embarrass me and I am ashamed to be around them.

2. Brainstorm options for protecting yourself. Below are some ways that Greg thought of to practice identity protection.

TYPES OF IDENTITY PROTECTION	GREG'S EXAMPLES
Cope with emotional stress In what ways can you take care of yourself as you heal from any emotional impacts that occur from your negative identity self-talk?	I am actually feeling mostly okay right now. But just in case, I could make sure I keep filling my wellness buckets [see page 114]—even though I may get judged for how I do so.
Filter social messages Are there any social messages about your racial and cultural background that are contributing to your negative identity self-talk? What kinds of information can you gather to help you determine if these social messages are true and helpful representations of your community?	I guess the stereotype that Latinos are only "true" Latinos if they like Reggaeton, Bachata, or something like that. I actually do listen to these types of music, but I also listen to other stuff. I mean there are Latino artists in other music genres who are really successful. So, am I supposed to think they aren't true Latinos? That's bogus.
Filter identity self-talk Are you noticing yourself accepting your negative identity self-talk as complete fact? What kinds of information can you gather to help you determine if such self-talk is a true and accurate representation of how you think and feel about your background?	I mean what does "acting White" even mean, though? I agree that not a lot of Latinos in my community like some of the things I like. Also, people really do think that only one type of person can like certain things. But I am trying to remember this doesn't mean I don't love or appreciate my Latino background and community. Being Latino isn't just a type of music or career. It's way more than that.
Grow my positive identity self-talk How can you continue making efforts to grow your self-love, self-confidence, and cultural pride with **identity exploration?** How can you continue making efforts to grow your self-love, self-confidence, and cultural pride with **identity expression?**	Identity exploration efforts could be remembering to step back and think about what being Latino really means to me. I recently learned there are more and more Latinos in STEM [science, technology, engineering, and mathematics]. I guess I could reach out to a few of them at the local community college and see what it's like to be around them. For me, my identity expression efforts will be to keep doing what I do. I just have to keep loving on my family and finding people who support me for me.

3. Create an identity protection plan. As you can imagine, negative identity self-talk can be very believable and become very distracting. Fortunately, Greg was able to use the steps in this chapter to:

- Come up with ways to take some mental steps back from his negative self-talk.
- Identify factual inaccuracies within his self-talk and the social messages connected with his self-talk.

That is, although he didn't necessary kick out the uninvited thought of "I am acting too White," he was able to identify why this thought is not a good representation of himself and find ways to continue building his positive identity self-talk while living alongside this thought. Hopefully Greg's use of these steps highlights some helpful ways for you to practice identity protection.

DESCRIBE YOUR EFFORT	WHEN DO YOU WANT TO PRACTICE?
IDENTITY PROTECTION EFFORT 1 Filter social messages	I plan to take a picture of the filter social messages questions and look at those questions anytime I am reminded of stereotypes about Latinos.
IDENTITY PROTECTION EFFORT 2 Grow my positive identity self-talk	I want to reach out to the leader of the Latino STEM club at my local community college and see if I could join one of their events before I enroll at the school.
IDENTITY PROTECTION EFFORT 3 Cope with emotional stress	I want to keep filling all my wellness buckets, but particularly my fun/enjoyment and accomplished/mastery buckets. I guess those kind of help me with my emotions and help me do things that make me feel good about being me.

YOUR TURN

Use the steps below to help you find the identity protection efforts that you can use to manage the impact of any negative identity self-talk you are experiencing.

1. Notice your negative identity self-talk. Describe the impact of your negative identity self-talk in the moment by answering the questions in the **Impacts of My Negative Identity Self-Talk worksheet** on the next page.

Impacts of My Negative Identity Self-Talk

THINGS TO THINK ABOUT	MY RESPONSES
What negative identity self-talk are you focusing on?	
Is this self-talk causing you any **emotional stress** in this moment?	o Yes o No o Somewhat
Explain your answer.	
Is this self-talk impacting your **self-love** in this moment?	o Yes o No o Somewhat
Explain your answer.	
Is this self-talk impacting your **self-confidence** in this moment?	o Yes o No o Somewhat
Explain your answer.	
Is this self-talk impacting your **cultural pride** in this moment?	o Yes o No o Somewhat
Explain your answer:	

2. Brainstorm options for protecting yourself. Now brainstorm options for protecting your self-love, self-confidence, and cultural pride. Try to think of at least three options for each category using the following worksheet.

My Options for Protecting Myself

Coping with emotional stress

What are three ways you could cope with any emotional stress associated with your negative identity self-talk?

1.

2.

3.

Filtering my self-talk

What are three ways you can check how true and accurate your self-talk is?

1.

2.

3.

Filtering social messages

What are three ways you can check the truth and accuracy of any social messages related to your self-talk?

1.

2.

3.

Growing my positive identity self-talk

What are three ways you can continue making efforts to grow your self-love, self-confidence, and cultural pride—despite having this negative identity self-talk?

1.

2.

3.

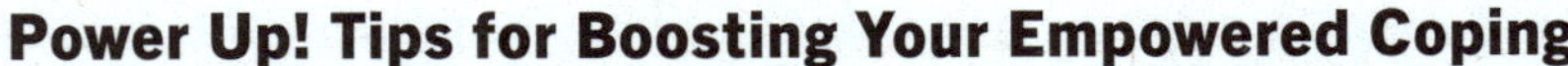

Power Up! Tips for Boosting Your Empowered Coping

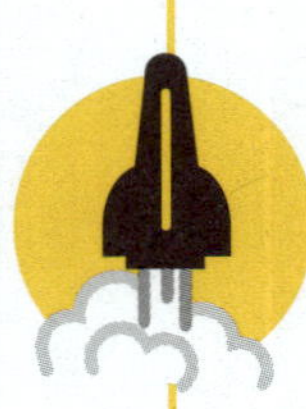

- **Start with emotional stress coping.** It can be extremely hard to use the filter questions and focus on growing your positive identity self-talk when experiencing strong and uncomfortable emotions. So, I encourage you to prioritize at least one emotional stress coping skill from Part Two in your brainstorming. Possibly consider a soothing effort from Chapter 8 or an option for filling a wellness bucket from Chapter 9 to help you manage the momentary or lingering emotional impacts of your negative identity self-talk.
- **Use the negative identity self-talk "things to think about" questions.** If you encounter difficulty filtering social messages or identity self-talk, try using the filter question tip sheet (pages 243–244) or look back at the worksheet on page 246 and consider your answers to the reflection prompts in the "Types of Identity Protection" column.
- **Calling in your workbook navigators:** Consider completing step 2 with one of your workbook navigators.

3. **Create an identity protection plan.** Now it's time to choose a few identity protection efforts to put into practice. List at least three identity protection efforts you're willing to put into action (in the worksheet on the facing page) and then set specific goals for when you will practice each effort.

Power Up! Tips for Boosting Your Empowered Coping

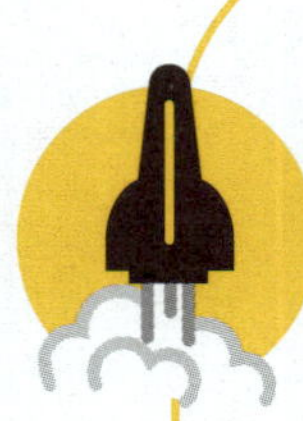

Before putting your plan into action, take a quick look at the reflection questions in the **Recap and Reflect** at the end of this chapter. Try to keep these questions in mind as you practice identity protection. Doing so will help you gather information to answer each prompt!

My Identity Protection Plan

DESCRIBE YOUR EFFORT	WHEN DO YOU WANT TO PRACTICE?
IDENTITY PROTECTION EFFORT 1	
IDENTITY PROTECTION EFFORT 2	
IDENTITY PROTECTION EFFORT 3	

Chapter 20: Recap and Reflect

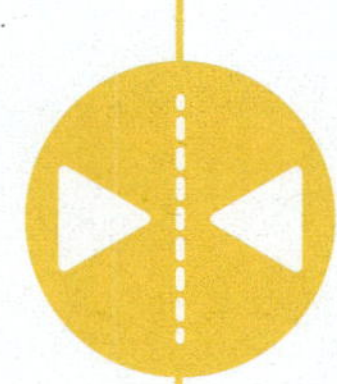

RECAP

- **Identity protection** describes our efforts to shield ourselves from any negative identity self-talk that lingers from culturally stressful events we have faced.
- The steps for practicing the identity protection skill include:
  1. Clarify the impact of negative identity self-talk.
  2. Brainstorm options for protecting yourself.
  3. Create an identity protection plan.

REFLECT

Hopefully you've had an opportunity to practice using your identity protection plan. Before moving forward, take a moment to think about what you learned about identity protection and how you hope to use this skill to cope with identity stress. To do so, answer the questions below.

Calling in your workbook navigators: You may also find it helpful to review your answers to these questions with your workbook navigators, as you may learn some new ways to put these coping decisions into action!

Which emotional stress coping skills have been most helpful when you've felt emotionally upset by negative identity self-talk?

Did you think of any extra filter questions that also help protect you from negative identity self-talk (and any social messages connected to your self-talk)?

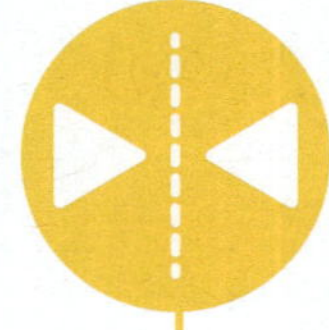

Despite experiencing negative identity self-talk, what ways have you been able to continue making efforts to grow your positive self-talk? Have any of your efforts helped you increase your self-love, self-confidence, or cultural pride?

PART FOUR SUMMARY AND TAKEAWAYS

- **Identity stress** describes instances when you struggle to experience self-love, self-confidence, and cultural pride before, during, or after a culturally stressful event.
- In Chapter 15 you learned how to notice the moments when you experience identity stress. Specifically, you learned to practice **mindfulness** by using the BEAT diagram to notice any positive or negative identity self-talk you have during your most culturally mindful moments.
- In Chapter 16 you learned that you may struggle to understand why you experience the types of negative identity self-talk you experience. To help you navigate this, **self-compassion** can help you show understanding toward the ways the social messages around you impact your identity self-talk.
- Chapter 17 introduced skills for building and maintaining your self-love, self-confidence, and cultural pride: identity exploration, identity expression, and

identity protection. You had a chance to assess which of these skills you have already been practicing and any that you want to strengthen by reading Chapters 18, 19, or 20.

- In Chapter 18 you learned that you can grow your self-love, self-confidence, and cultural pride by taking time to clarify the parts of your background you feel most connected to. Specifically, you practiced using **identity exploration** to discover who you are and how you want to express this part of your identity.
- In Chapter 19 you learned that you can grow your self-love, self-confidence, and cultural pride by finding spaces to confidently and authentically express your background. Specifically, you practiced using **identity expression** to help you identify where you feel most comfortable being your authentic self and created a plan to build your emotional tolerance for self-expression.
- In Chapter 20 you learned that identity stress can occur when you don't know how to manage the impact of your negative identity self-talk. To help you navigate this, you need your **identity protection skills** to help you build and protect your self-love, self-confidence, and cultural pride.

TRACK YOUR IDENTITY STRESS COPING

Whenever you notice yourself experiencing identity stress when facing a culturally stressful event, keep track of what empowered coping decisions you make to build and protect your self-love, self-confidence, and cultural pride. In the following worksheet, write the date when you noticed the identity stress and then describe whether you used any coping skills from Chapter 16 (**self-compassion**), Chapter 18 (**identity exploration**), Chapter 19 (**identity expression**), or Chapter 20 (**identity protection**). Also, there is a column for any empowered coping decisions you make that don't fall into these four categories.

My Identity Stress Coping

NOTICED IDENTITY STRESS	SELF-COMPASSION	IDENTITY EXPLORATION	IDENTITY EXPRESSION	IDENTITY PROTECTION	OTHER IDENTITY STRESS COPING
Date:					
Date:					
Date:					
Date:					
Date:					
Date:					

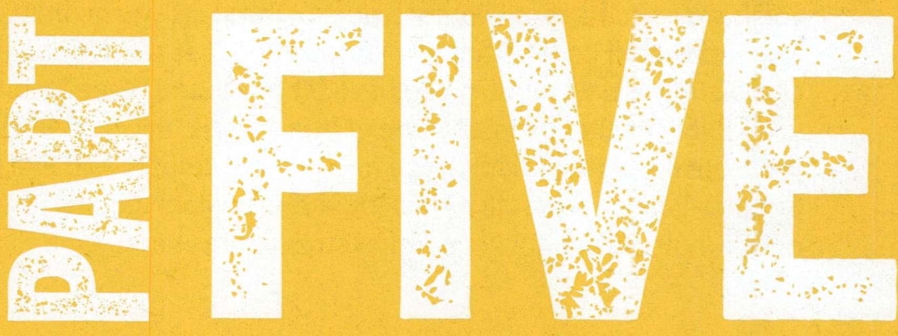

PART FIVE

Putting the Pieces of Empowered Coping Together!

The final section of this book will help you pause and practice putting together all you have learned about yourself and all the skills you've built. Below are the steps for empowered coping that you learned about at the very beginning of this book. By completing this workbook, you have bit by bit and piece by piece been strengthening your ability to engage in all three of these steps. In Chapter 21, you will summarize all you've learned that enables you to complete steps 1 and 2 of empowered coping. In Chapter 22, you'll practice thinking through which coping skills to prioritize when you notice multiple impacts of cultural stress at the same time.

EMPOWERED COPING

1. **Clarifying the impact of cultural stress:** Has this event or situation caused you emotional stress, agency stress, or identity stress?
2. **Think of what "I can" do:** Which of your abilities and resources can you use to cope with the stress you are experiencing?
3. **Make empowered coping decisions:** How can you use your abilities and resources to make the best decision for you in this moment and moving forward?

21 How Do I Remember Everything I've Learned?

In this chapter, you're going to describe what helps you notice the cultural stress impacts you're experiencing and list the coping skills you can use for each. To summarize your learning and serve as a handy tool for quick reference, you will create a **cultural stress coping card** for each cultural stress impact: emotional, agency, and identity stress. First you'll see how our navigators completed their coping cards, and then you'll have a chance to complete your own.

Power Up! Tips for Boosting Your Empowered Coping

You may find it helpful to look back at your responses in Parts Two, Three, and Four of the workbook to help complete your cards. This review will ensure you don't omit any of what you've learned.

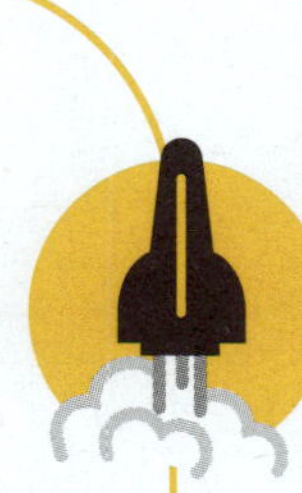

CREATING YOUR EMOTIONAL STRESS COPING CARD

As you learned in Part Two, **emotional stress** describes moments when we experience uncomfortable body sensations and emotions when faced with culturally stressful events. In Chapter 4 you learned to use the BEAT diagram and the emotional stress zones chart to help you identify which body sensations and emotions are the strongest signs that you've been impacted emotionally by a culturally stressful experience. Then you learned to use each of the emotional stress coping skills listed in the diagram below. You're going to summarize everything you've learned about riding the wave of emotional stress in one coping card. First, take a look at how Amia created her emotional stress coping card.

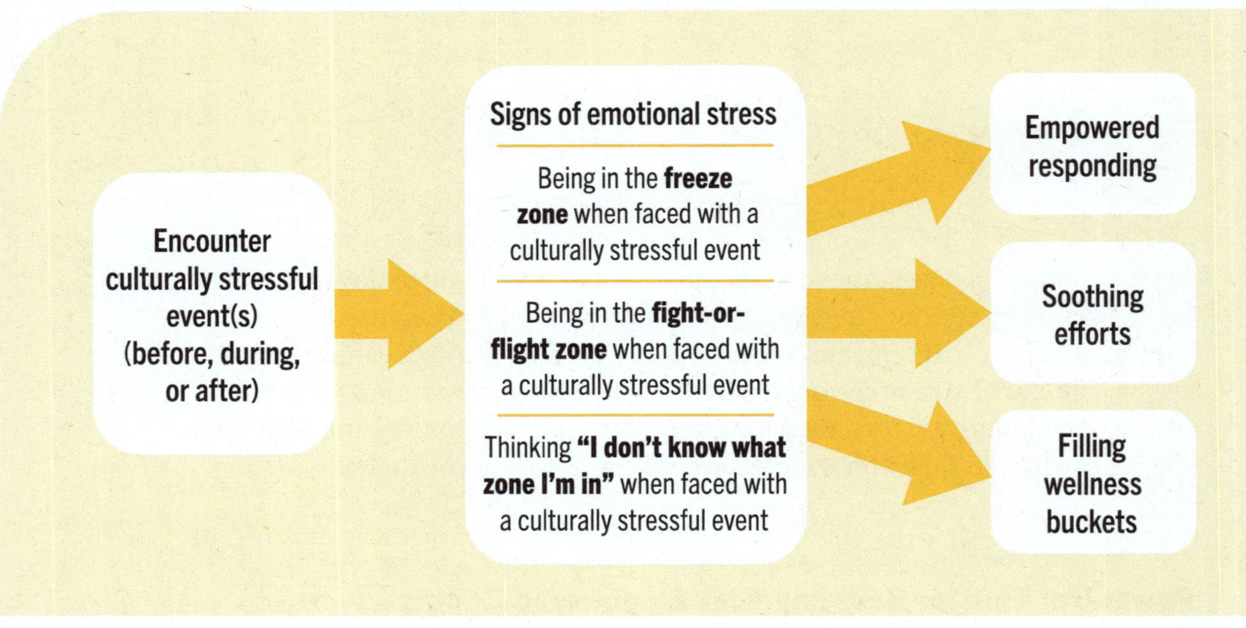

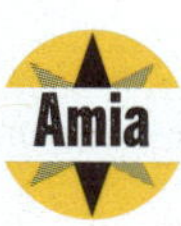

Amia's Emotional Stress Coping Card

EMOTIONAL STRESS COPING TARGETS	MY EMPOWERED COPING SKILLS
Mindfulness What *can* I look for in my **BEAT diagram** to help me notice emotional stress?	**Body sensations:** - Feeling sweaty; uncomfortable stomach **Emotions:** - Feeling intense anxiety and fear **Action/urges:** - Wanting to avoid people/places; wanting to hide who I am **Thoughts:** - Noticing thoughts like "If I bring attention to myself, people will tease me"
Self-compassion When I notice emotional stress, I *can* **show kindness and understanding** toward my emotions by:	- Noticing that I often use a lot of <u>should</u> thoughts to judge myself, like "I shouldn't have cried in front of him" - Now I try to say, "I notice I am feeling nervous and upset, but this makes sense for me in this situation because . . ."
Empowered responding When I notice emotional stress, I *can* **make helpful decisions in the moment** by:	- Noticing I typically want to avoid or escape situations - Trying to think carefully about when and why I should practice empowered responding to help me go or stay somewhere that makes me feel nervous - I have learned to use some of my values in my Who Am I? diagram to help me make these decisions. I ask myself if avoiding people/places is taking me closer or further away from what I care about most in life.
Soothing efforts When I notice emotional stress, I *can* **soothe my emotions** by:	- Controlled breathing works best for me. Then I can use listening to music, going for walks, and prayer as my calming activities. - I am still growing in my seeking social support. I have one friend at my mosque that I have talked to about my emotions and will try to keep doing so.
Filling wellness buckets When I notice emotional stress, I *can* **make healthy decisions over time** as I heal by:	- Making sure I keep filling my social connection bucket—especially the ones outside of my school - Making sure I keep filling my accomplishment/mastery bucket by continuing to work hard in school

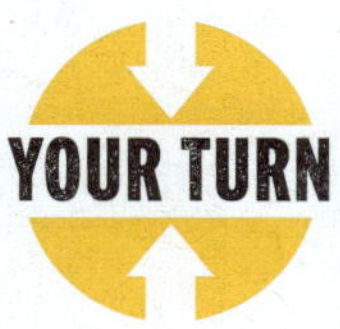

Use the worksheet on the next page to complete your **emotional stress coping card.** Feel free to look back over your responses in Part Two to help you fill in your coping card.

My Emotional Stress Coping Card

EMOTIONAL STRESS COPING TARGETS	MY EMPOWERED COPING SKILLS
Mindfulness What *can* I look for in my **BEAT diagram** to help me notice emotional stress?	**Body sensations:** **Emotions:** **Action/urges:** **Thoughts:**
Self-compassion When I notice emotional stress, I *can* **show kindness and understanding** toward my emotions by:	
Empowered responding When I notice emotional stress, I *can* **make helpful decisions in the moment** by:	
Soothing efforts When I notice emotional stress, I *can* **soothe my emotions** by:	
Filling wellness buckets When I notice emotional stress, I *can* **make healthy decisions over time** as I heal by:	
When I notice emotional stress, I *can* also (describe any other coping skills you can use):	

CREATING YOUR AGENCY STRESS COPING CARD

You learned in Part Three that **agency stress** describes the moments when you feel a low sense of control over your culturally stressful surroundings. In Chapter 10, you learned that "I can't" thinking, avoiding change efforts, and feeling dissatisfied with the outcome of your change efforts can be signs of agency stress within your BEAT diagram. Then you learned to use both of the agency stress coping skills listed in the diagram below. Just as you did with emotional stress, I invite you to create a coping card that summarizes all you can do when faced with agency stress. First, see how Jamal created his agency stress coping card.

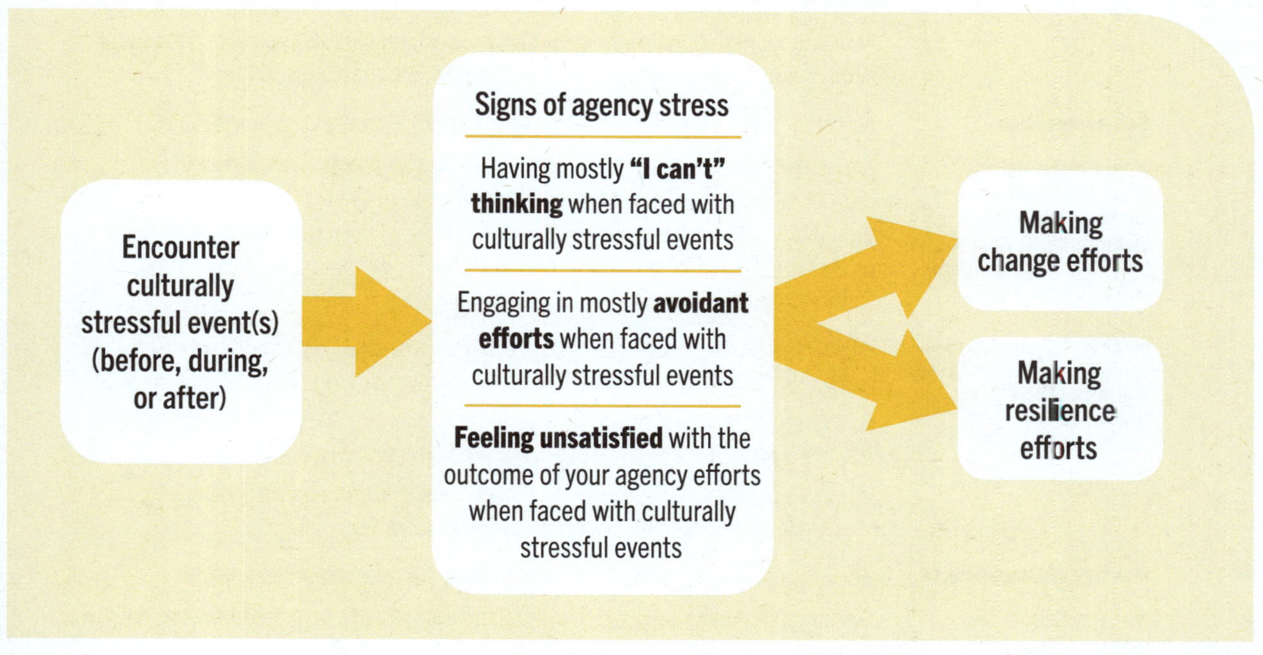

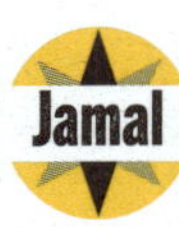

Jamal's Agency Stress Coping Card

AGENCY STRESS COPING TARGETS	MY EMPOWERED COPING SKILLS
Mindfulness What *can* I look for in my **BEAT diagram** to help me notice agency stress?	**Body sensations:** - Feeling exhausted or worn down **Emotions:** - Feeling hopeless and sad **Action/urges:** - Noticing avoidant efforts, like strong urges to quit my job or spending hours researching other jobs instead of focusing on my work at this job **Thoughts:** - Noticing "I can't" thinking like "I can't say anything to check my boss" or "I can't say or do anything to achieve my career goals, like getting promoted"
Self-compassion When I notice agency stress, I *can* **show kindness and understanding** toward how I handle any culturally stressful events by:	- Noticing I tend to self-blame when upset about my change efforts - Remembering to both acknowledge my coping challenges and others' responsibility—this helps me reduce some of my self-blame - Also, acknowledging my learning has helped me get unstuck from my "I can't" mindset; it helps me begin brainstorming what "I can" do the next time I am in a situation
Making change efforts When I notice agency stress, I *can* pursue my **change goals** by:	- Trying to keep my boundaries clear with my colleagues when I am willing to accept any costs that may come from this (confront and communicate) - Educating my colleagues about my experience when I am willing to accept any costs that may come from this (confront and communicate) - Joining a professional organization that allows me to support the next generation of Black professionals (engage in activism)
Making resilience efforts When I notice agency stress, I *can* use these **resilience efforts** to pursue my goals by: I *can* also use these **supportive actions** to navigate any cultural stress that may get in the way of my resilience efforts:	- Showing up to my job daily and working hard on my assigned projects - Signing up for work projects that expand my skill sets and that prepare me for advancement in this job (or elsewhere) - Continuing to learn who I can trust in this job (information seeking) - Keeping to my work schedule and trying not to work too late (selective energy and effort) - Building new relationships with Black professionals while maintaining connections with my college friends (maintaining supportive networks)

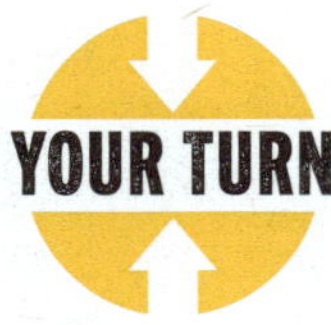

Use the table on the facing page to fill in complete your **agency stress coping card.** Feel free to look back over your responses in Part Three to help you fill in your coping card.

My Agency Stress Coping Card

AGENCY STRESS COPING TARGETS	MY EMPOWERED COPING SKILLS
Mindfulness What *can* I look for in my **BEAT diagram** to help me notice agency stress?	**Body sensations:** **Emotions:** **Action/urges:** **Thoughts:**
Self-compassion When I notice agency stress, I *can* **show kindness and understanding** toward how I handle any culturally stressful events by:	
Making change efforts When I notice agency stress, I *can* pursue my **change goals** by:	
Making resilience efforts When I notice agency stress, I *can* use these **resilience efforts** to pursue my goals by: I *can* also use these **supportive actions** to navigate any cultural stress that may get in the way of my resilience efforts:	
When I notice agency stress, I *can* also (describe any other coping skills you can use):	

CREATING YOUR IDENTITY STRESS COPING CARD

You learned in Part Four that **identity stress** describes instances when you struggle to experience positive identity self-talk (self-love, self-confidence, and cultural pride) before, during, or after a culturally stressful event. In Chapter 15, you learned to use your BEAT diagram to be on the lookout for any negative identity self-talk (self-dislike, self-doubt, or cultural shame) that may result from experiences with cultural stress. Then you learned to use each of the identity stress coping skills listed in the diagram below. Here you're invited to create an identity stress coping card that summarizes all you can do to either strengthen your positive identity self-talk or protect you from any lingering negative identity self-talk. First, take a look at how Greg created his coping card.

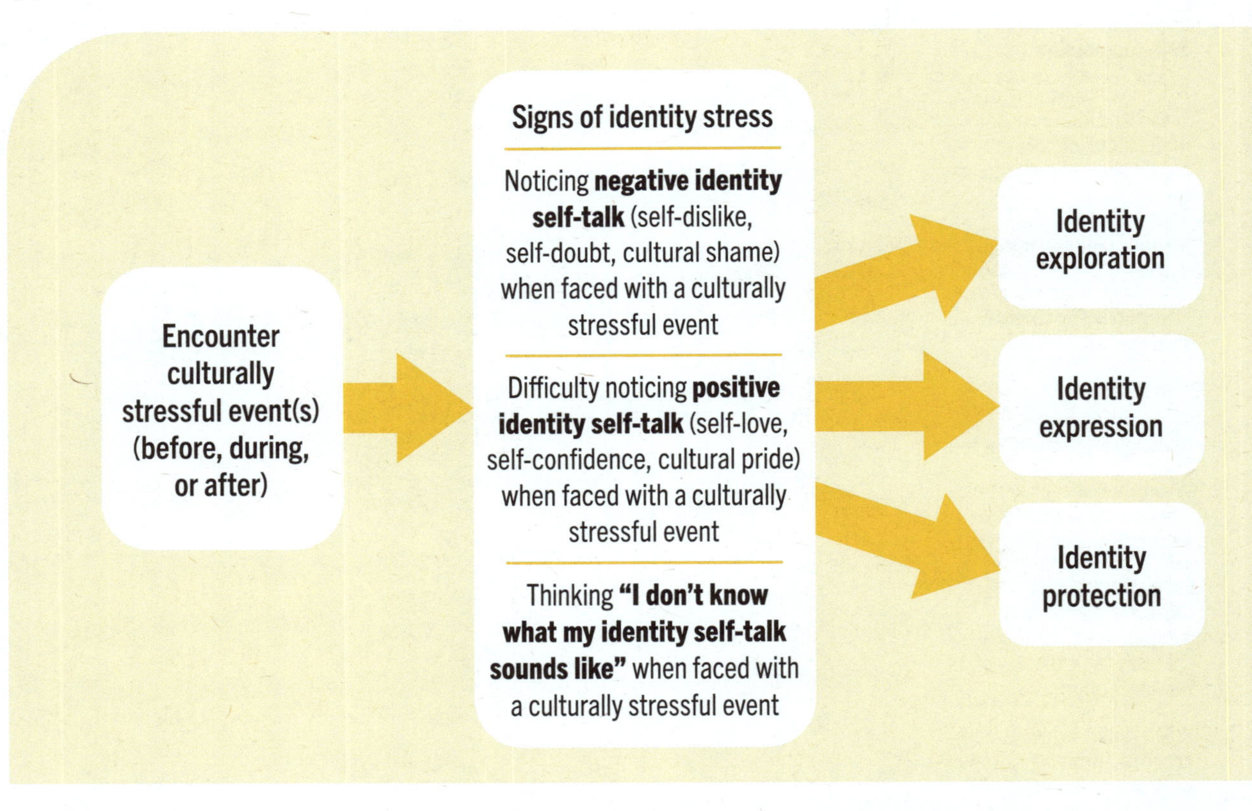

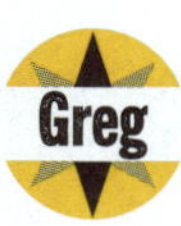

Greg's Identity Stress Coping Card

IDENTITY STRESS COPING TARGETS	MY EMPOWERED COPING SKILLS
Mindfulness What *can* I look for in my **BEAT diagram** to help me notice identity stress?	**Body sensations:** - Feeling tense in my muscles **Emotions:** - Feeling shame and embarrassment **Action/urges:** - Hiding my thoughts, opinions, and interests from people **Thoughts:** - Noticing self-dislike thinking, like "I am acting too White"
Self-compassion When I notice identity stress, I *can* **show kindness and understanding** toward my identity self-talk by:	- Reminding myself about the stereotypes that people use to judge and criticize Latinos - Reminding myself that it makes sense that sometimes I may question who I am if I am surrounded by people who judge and treat me differently based on these stereotypes - Reminding myself that having these thoughts doesn't mean they are true and doesn't mean I don't love my community
Identity exploration When I notice identity stress, I *can* still **explore and discover** what I love and appreciate about my identity by:	- Remembering to practice identity exploration regularly and not just when experiencing cultural stress - I want to keep reading about Latinos in STEM, learning about types of Latino musicians who play nontraditional styles of music, and maybe even interview my family members about our family's history.
Identity expression When I notice identity stress, I *can* still find ways to **confidently express** my identity by:	- Continuing to listen to the types of music I enjoy, spending time with my family, continuing to speak Spanish with my family and in my community, and attending cultural events that fully celebrate Latine culture (not just what my friends celebrate) - Finding more places to openly express myself outside my friend group - Setting a goal to at least selectively express myself around my friends instead of not sharing anything about myself or acting as if I like certain things that I really don't
Identity protection When I notice identity stress, I *can* **protect** my self-love, self-confidence, and cultural pride by:	- Using the filtering social messages questions from the tip sheet - Focusing on growing my positive identity self-talk by focusing on the above identity exploration and expression efforts - Remembering to cope with any emotional stress caused by my negative identity self-talk by using the skills in my emotional stress coping card

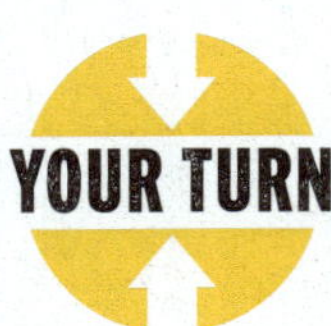

Use the worksheet on the facing page to complete your **identity stress coping card.** Feel free to look back over your responses in Part Four to help you fill in your coping card.

Chapter 21: Recap and Reflect

RECAP

- **Cultural stress coping cards** are a memory tool that can help you quickly recall the coping skills you can use when experiencing emotional stress, agency stress, or identity stress.
- As a refresher, **emotional stress coping** includes the following skills: mindfulness, self-compassion, empowered responding, soothing efforts, and filling wellness buckets.
- **Agency stress coping** includes the following skills: mindfulness, self-compassion, making change efforts, and making resilience efforts.
- **Identity stress coping** includes the following skills: mindfulness, self-compassion, identity exploration, identity expression, and identity protection.

REFLECT

You have just created your cultural stress coping cards! Doing so is a sign of all the hard work you have put into completing this workbook. Now take a few moments and use the prompts below to reflect on how you can maximize your use of the coping cards.

What can you do to keep easy access to your cultural stress coping cards?

As you grow and your surroundings change, you will likely need to update your coping cards. What are some signs that you may need or want to update your cultural stress coping cards?

Are you willing to share your cultural stress coping cards with any of your workbook navigators? If so, which of your workbook navigators are you willing to share your coping cards with?

My Identity Stress Coping Card

IDENTITY STRESS COPING TARGETS	MY EMPOWERED COPING SKILLS
Mindfulness What *can* I look for in my **BEAT diagram** to help me notice identity stress?	**Body sensations:** **Emotions:** **Action/urges:** **Thoughts:**
Self-compassion When I notice identity stress, I *can* **show kindness and understanding** toward my identity self-talk by:	
Identity exploration When I notice identity stress, I *can* still **explore and discover** what I love and appreciate about my identity by:	
Identity expression When I notice identity stress, I *can* still find ways to **confidently express** my identity by:	
Identity protection When I notice identity stress, I *can* **protect** my self-love, self-confidence, and cultural pride by:	
When I notice identity stress, I *can* also (describe any other coping skills you can use):	

22 How Can I Use My Cultural Stress Coping Cards to Practice Empowered Coping?

Rarely do culturally stressful events impact you in only one way. You're likely, in fact, to experience all three impacts at the same time, which can make coping with cultural stress much more difficult. That's why learning to practice step 3 of the empowered coping steps (shown below) is so important. This chapter will help you strengthen your ability to select the tools from your cultural stress coping cards that are the best fit for the stressful moment you are in.

EMPOWERED COPING
1. **Clarifying the impact of cultural stress:** Has this event or situation caused you emotional stress, agency stress, or identity stress?
2. **Think of what "I can" do:** Which of your abilities and resources can you use to cope with the stress you are experiencing?
3. **Make empowered coping decisions:** How can you use your abilities and resources to make the best decision for you in this moment and moving forward?

Before you choose your own coping skills, let's see how Jamal puts all the pieces of the empowered coping steps together. As you may recall from Chapter 3, Jamal experienced several culturally stressful events from the time he walked to work until he left to go home. The following table summarizes the impacts these events had on him.

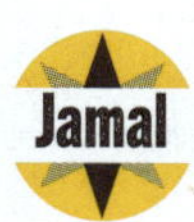

Jamal's Cultural Stress

TYPE OF STRESS	THE IMPACTS OF JAMAL'S CULTURAL STRESS EVENTS
Emotional stress	Jamal felt annoyed, hopeless, and ultimately exhausted by his work experiences.
Agency stress	When asked to take the lead on a committee focused on police brutality, Jamal felt he couldn't say no to his boss without suffering unwanted consequences.
Identity stress	After learning about the academic connection his White colleagues had with their boss, Jamal thought, "There's no way someone like me would ever be considered [for the promotion]."

Completing this workbook helped Jamal realize that on that single Monday he had experienced all three cultural stress impacts. Take a look at how he decided which impacts to prioritize coping with on that day. Then you can practice putting all the empowered coping steps together for a culturally stressful event you've experienced.

1. **Notice the impact of cultural stress.** Here is where the mindfulness skills you've been strengthening come into the picture. As you've done throughout this workbook, you start with pausing and describing your BEAT reactions to a culturally stressful event. Jamal used the worksheet below to help him complete step 1 of the empowered coping steps.

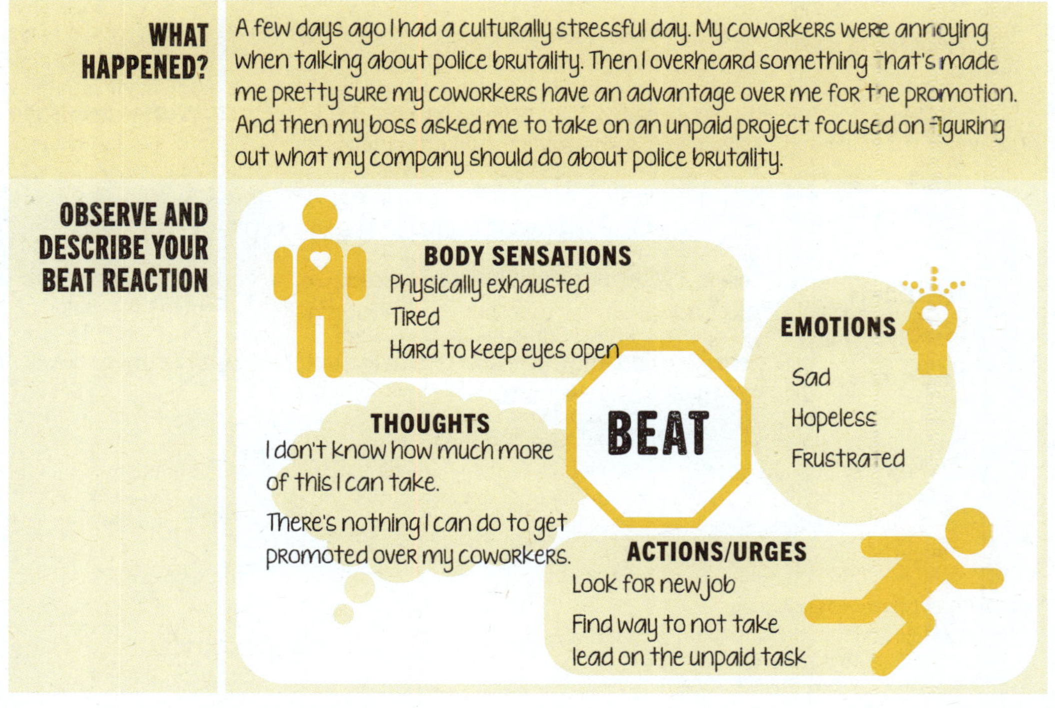

NOTICING YOUR CULTURAL STRESS IMPACTS		
	Emotional stress: Are you noticing any strong and uncomfortable body sensations or emotions in this moment?	● Yes ○ No
	Agency stress: Are you noticing avoidance urges, "I can't" thoughts, or dissatisfaction in your change efforts that are making it hard to feel a sense of control in this moment?	● Yes ○ No
	Identity stress: Are you noticing negative identity self-talk that's making it hard to experience self-love, self-confidence, or cultural pride in this moment?	● Yes ○ No

2. Think of what you can do. Next it's time to see what you have in your toolkit to help you cope with the cultural stress impacts you're experiencing. On the facing page is the **Empowered Coping Decision Tree,** which summarizes Parts Two through Four of this workbook in one diagram. You may find it helpful to use this decision tree to choose which cultural stress coping cards you want to look over in the moment you are in. If you ever struggle to know which cultural stress impacts to focus on first, see the Tip Sheet on pages 272–273 for some ideas.

Whichever cultural stress impacts you decide to focus on, try to identify at least three to five skills from your coping cards that you can put into action. Below are the skills Jamal considered using after his stressful workday.

I could try to . . .	Show kindness and understanding toward my BEAT by thinking about how my emotions make sense given what all happened.
I could try to . . .	Use the soothing efforts from my emotional stress coping card and try to stick to my wellness plan.
I could try to . . .	Keep making resilience efforts toward my career goals at work (at least until I decide whether I truly want to stay at this job or not).
I could try to . . .	Connect with one of my Black senior-level coworkers and see if they might have some advice on how to pursue my career goals.
I could try to . . .	Keep up my identity expression efforts to protect against any negative identity self-talk linked to that day.

Empowered Coping Decision Tree

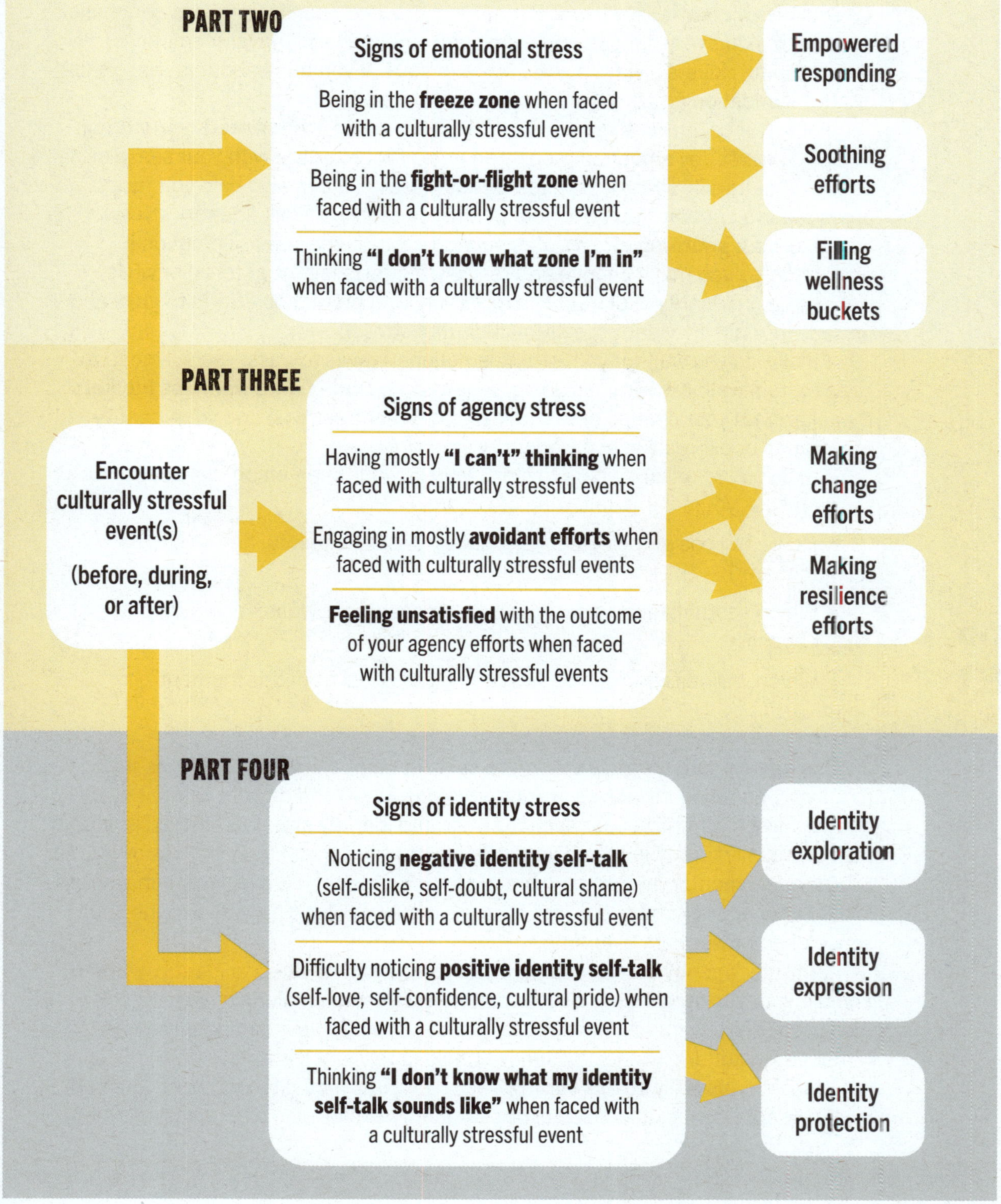

Encounter culturally stressful event(s)

(before, during, or after)

PART TWO

Signs of emotional stress

- Being in the **freeze zone** when faced with a culturally stressful event
- Being in the **fight-or-flight zone** when faced with a culturally stressful event
- Thinking **"I don't know what zone I'm in"** when faced with a culturally stressful event

→ Empowered responding
→ Soothing efforts
→ Filling wellness buckets

PART THREE

Signs of agency stress

- Having mostly **"I can't" thinking** when faced with culturally stressful events
- Engaging in mostly **avoidant efforts** when faced with culturally stressful events
- **Feeling unsatisfied** with the outcome of your agency efforts when faced with culturally stressful events

→ Making change efforts
→ Making resilience efforts

PART FOUR

Signs of identity stress

- Noticing **negative identity self-talk** (self-dislike, self-doubt, cultural shame) when faced with a culturally stressful event
- Difficulty noticing **positive identity self-talk** (self-love, self-confidence, cultural pride) when faced with a culturally stressful event
- Thinking **"I don't know what my identity self-talk sounds like"** when faced with a culturally stressful event

→ Identity exploration
→ Identity expression
→ Identity protection

Tip Sheet: Knowing Where to Focus Your Empowered Coping Efforts

1. Start with emotional stress. Because strong and intense emotions can make decision making very difficult and even confusing, focusing on your emotional stress coping skills is always a good place to start. If you think about it, these skills are the foundation for all the other skills we've discussed.

For instance, strengthening your ability to practice **empowered responding** helps you resist any emotionally charged urges that interfere with your sense of control in culturally stressful spaces (agency stress). It can also help you resist urges that do not help you build your positive identity self-talk (identity stress).

Also, your **soothing efforts** offer you tools to ride the wave of emotional discomfort as you make change and resilience efforts (agency stress) or while you engage in identity exploration, expression, and protection efforts to grow and protect your positive identity self-talk (identity stress).

Finally, as you wait for your strong emotional waves to pass, you still need to keep certain wellness routines going, which can include **filling wellness buckets** that align with your change or resilience goals (agency stress) and your identity exploration or expression goals (identity stress).

So, if you are unsure where to start, lean on your three emotional stress coping skills and ask yourself the following questions.

- How can I use empowered responding to make a helpful decision in this moment?
- Which soothing efforts can I use while engaging in whatever action plan I choose?
- Which wellness buckets do I want to fill as I heal from this moment?

2. Use agency and identity coping to sustain empowerment. However, if you focus only on riding the waves of your emotions day in and day out without ever finding ways to prioritize your agency stress and identity stress coping skills, you may eventually grow weary and your coping efforts may feel meaningless over time. So, in the moments when you are not experiencing all-consuming emotional stress, look to your agency stress or identity stress coping skills as ways to expand your sense of empowerment over time.

Consider **agency stress coping** if you feel most motivated to identify ways to change your surroundings to be less culturally stressful (making change efforts). Also use it if you want to identify goals you can still pursue meaningfully while remaining in culturally stressful spaces (making resilience efforts).

Consider **identity stress coping** if you feel most motivated to boost your self-love, self-confidence, and cultural pride (identity exploration or expression). Also use it if you need to protect yourself from any lingering negative identity self-talk (identity protection).

If unsure which of these coping options would be best to prioritize, look to your BEAT diagram to notice which signs of agency or identity stress are most bothersome in that moment.

3. Don't forget about self-compassion. It is a natural human desire to look at coping as only a set of strategies to fix a problem. However, cultural stress is not a problem that comes with an easy fix or a quick resolution. Rather, it's more like a problem that pops up and shows itself again and again over time. So, regardless of what empowered coping skills you put into action, don't forget to show kindness and understanding toward yourself. Despite your best and most thoughtful efforts to implement the skills in this workbook, experience says you will feel emotional pain again. You will again be in a situation where you feel a lack of control. And you will have moments when your self-talk isn't the kindest and most affirming. When these things happen, you may be tempted to say, "I am not doing this right" or "See, I knew I couldn't feel more empowered." The constant references to self-compassion throughout this workbook were made intentionally to serve as a reminder to be kind and understanding toward yourself as you make your best efforts to navigate the challenging task of coping with cultural stress. Because such coping is not simple and is an ever-evolving process, remember to keep your compassionate narrator close by—especially when you feel as if your coping efforts are falling short. Doing so will help you stay on or find your path back to empowered coping.

3. Make an empowered coping decision. Now it's time to put into action your best coping options. In the worksheet below, **primary empowered coping decisions** are the skills you feel are most important to prioritize. **Secondary empowered coping decisions** are the skills you know are important for building a sense of empowerment over time but you feel they are best to engage in only once your emotional stress is somewhat reduced. Below are the coping decisions Jamal chose to put into action.

PRIMARY EMPOWERED COPING DECISIONS	**I want to prioritize:** showing kindness and understanding toward my BEAT, using my soothing efforts, and sticking to my wellness plan.
SECONDARY EMPOWERED COPING DECISIONS	**Eventually I want to make sure I also:** clarify the resilience goals I feel most motivated to keep pursuing and reach out to the senior-level coworker. I'll also try to make at least one identity expression effort before the end of the week

Ultimately, Jamal hoped that focusing on the emotional stress coping skills for a few days would help him attain some emotional relief before putting into action his secondary empowered coping decisions. So he practiced a few soothing efforts he learned in Chapter 8. Also, he made sure to focus on filling his physical wellness bucket, by keeping a consistent bedtime and working out daily, along with filling his social connection bucket, by texting a few friends and asking to hang out over the next few days. This plan seems to work well for Jamal at this moment. However, if you were in a situation similar to Jamal's, you might consider a different set of coping decisions—that's absolutely okay. Remember, the empowered coping steps are intended to help you expand your "I can" mindset and help you put into action the coping skills that give you the best chance to attain the coping goals you have for yourself.

FINAL ACTIVITY

And now for the finale! The goal of this final activity is for you to think of a current or anticipated culturally stressful event and practice the empowered coping steps from start to finish: pausing and noticing the impact of this event, brainstorming what you can do to cope, and then deciding which coping skills to put into action. Also, think of this activity as an exercise you can come back to whenever you encounter a culturally stressful event, as it will guide you through using everything you have learned from this workbook. Use the prompts to see what empowered coping decisions you come up with.

1. **Notice the impact of cultural stress.** Use the **Impact of a Culturally Stressful Event worksheet** (facing page) to help you complete step 1 of the empowered coping steps and clarify which cultural stress impacts to focus on in this moment.

2. **Think of what you can do.** Next, with the **Coping Skills I Can Try worksheet** (page 276), try to identify at least three to five skills that you can put into action. Remember, you can use the Empowered Coping Decision Tree (page 271) and your cultural stress coping cards (page 267) to help you think of the skills you have available to you.

3. **Make an empowered coping decision.** Finally, use **My Empowered Coping Priorities** (page 276) to pick and put into action your best coping options.

Impact of a Culturally Stressful Event

WHAT HAPPENED?

OBSERVE AND DESCRIBE YOUR BEAT REACTION

BODY SENSATIONS

EMOTIONS

THOUGHTS

BEAT

ACTIONS/URGES

NOTICE YOUR CULTURAL STRESS IMPACTS		
	Emotional stress: Are you noticing any strong and uncomfortable body sensations or emotions in this moment?	○ Yes ○ No
	Agency stress: Are you noticing avoidance urges, "I can't" thoughts, or dissatisfaction in your change efforts that are making it hard to feel a sense of control in this moment?	○ Yes ○ No
	Identity stress: Are you noticing negative identity self-talk that's making it hard to experience self-love, self-confidence, or cultural pride in this moment?	○ Yes ○ No

Coping Skills I Can Try

I could try to . . .	
I could try to . . .	
I could try to . . .	
I could try to . . .	
I could try to . . .	

My Empowered Coping Priorities

PRIMARY EMPOWERED COPING DECISIONS	**I want to prioritize:**
SECONDARY EMPOWERED COPING DECISIONS	**Eventually, I want to make sure I also:**

Chapter 22: Recap and Reflect

RECAP

- **Empowered coping** describes your ability to (1) clarify how cultural stress is impacting you, (2) identify what you can do to cope with its impacts, and (3) make the most empowered coping decision for you in a given moment.
- If unsure where to focus your empowered coping efforts, start with practicing your **emotional stress coping skills.**
- **Use agency and identity stress coping skills** to build and sustain a sense of empowerment over time
- **Don't forget about self-compassion.** This skill will help you be kind and understanding to yourself as you make your best efforts to navigate the challenging realities that complicate your cultural stress coping.

REFLECT

You now have all the tools to practice empowered coping whenever faced with culturally stressful events. When practicing empowered coping, it is always important to remember that there is no true right or wrong coping decision. Instead, the goal is to use the three empowered coping steps to find the coping decisions that work best for you. The final reflection takes you back to the beginning of your journey in this workbook. Revisit your Who Am I? diagram from Chapter 1 and consider which parts of this diagram can be used to help you make empowered coping decisions.

Which **values** from your Who Am I? diagram do you want to prioritize whenever you are practicing the empowered coping steps?

Which **personal abilities** from your Who Am I? diagram might be helpful to lean on whenever you are practicing the empowered coping steps?

Which **interests** from your Who Am I? diagram can you use to practice the empowered coping steps?

Conclusion

Continuing Your Empowered Coping Journey

Congrats! You have done the hard work of learning how culturally stressful events have impacted your life and then practiced using different coping skills to navigate and heal from these impacts. Your journey of learning is by no means over, but my hope is that you have grown a great deal during your completion of this workbook. As you move forward, keep these final tips in mind.

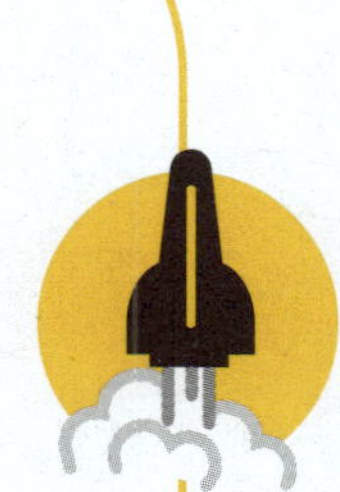

Power Up! Tips for Boosting Your Empowered Coping

- Remember to use your empowered coping steps when faced with a culturally stressful event.
- Keep your Cultural Stress Coping Cards close and accessible.
  - Put your completed cards on your smartphone for easy reference.
  - Carry a physical copy in your wallet (you can download and print them from the website).
  - Post your cards somewhere in your home where you'll see them often.
- Maintain connection with your workbook navigators.
- Revisit the contents of this workbook anytime you (or your workbook navigators) feel unsure how to identify an empowered coping decision.

Before we wrap up our time together, I want to say "Thank You!" again. I am truly honored that you decided to add this workbook to your coping toolkit. I hope the resources in this book have helped you deepen your self-love and helped you heal from the stressful events that brought you to this book. I generally wish you all the best in your continued empowered coping journey!

Therapy Resources

WHAT IS THERAPY?

Therapy, in this case specifically psychotherapy, is a form of health care in which a person discusses their concerns with a therapist and then receives different forms of support, such as:

- Validation and emotional support
- New perspectives on life
- A better understanding of oneself
- Gaining new skills for managing life's stresses

HOW DO I FIND A THERAPIST THAT WORKS FOR ME?

Many different factors are involved in finding a good fit with a therapist, such as:

- Do you prefer therapy meetings in person versus on video?
- Does the provider accept your insurance?
- Do you feel that the therapist has a good understanding of the symptoms you are experiencing?
- Do you get an overall "good vibe" from the therapist when you speak with them?

Other factors may impact your comfort with talking to a therapist as well. You might consider chatting with your workbook navigators about what they would look for in a therapist, or what those who have tried therapy looked for.

What might give you a "good vibe" about a particular therapist? For some, this assessment is heavily influenced by whether they feel their therapist is culturally attuned and respectful—meaning the therapist is affirming of their racial and cultural background and creates space for them to share any culturally stressful experiences they've had. Below are a few therapist directories that feature clinicians of color (many of which specialize in having supportive conversations about the cultural stresses covered in this book).

- Inclusive Therapists (*www.inclusivetherapists.com*), a directory focused on the needs/interests of persons of color and the LGBTQ community
- South Asian Therapists (*www.southasiantherapists.org*), a directory focused on the needs/interests of the South Asian diaspora
- Therapy for Black Girls (*www.therapyforblackgirls.com*), a directory focused on the needs/interests of Black women and girls
- Therapy for Black Men (*www.therapyforblackmen.org*), a directory focused on the needs/interests of Black men and boys
- Therapy for Latinx (*www.therapyforlatinx.com*), a directory focused on the needs/interests of the Latine community
- InnoPsych (*www.innopsych.com*), a directory focused on the needs/interests of persons of color

Unfortunately, at times it can be hard to find a therapist who shares a racial and cultural background with you. So your therapy options may include only therapists who do not share your background. If this is your situation, consider asking your prospective therapist for a brief consultation call and use some of the questions below to see if you'd feel comfortable speaking with them:

- Have you worked with people who wanted to better understand which parts of their racial and cultural background they feel most connected to?
- Have you worked with people who wanted to discuss concerns involving being treated differently due to their race, ethnicity, or cultural background?
- I have been struggling to cope with cultural stress in these ways: [describe your experience possibly using your responses to the Cultural Stress Impact Questionnaire in Chapter 3]. How have you helped or supported others who have had experiences similar to mine?
- My racial and cultural communities are [describe your responses in the "I am" section of your Who Am I? diagram on page 14]. I consider this an important part of my identity. Have you treated others who belong to these communities before?
- How do you try to show respect for someone's racial and cultural background in the therapy you offer?
- What kind of education or training have you had in providing culturally sensitive care?

From questions like these, you can hopefully get a sense of how comfortable, confident, and open a therapist might be in discussing topics related to cultural stress in your therapy.

Scholarly Inspirations

There are many scholars whose contributions to the field of mental health have greatly impacted my clinical practice. In an effort to celebrate the work of those who've inspired me, I've listed below the scholarly works that had the greatest influence on the design of this workbook. I am extremely grateful for the contributions of these scholars along with the work of countless others who paved the way for me as a Black psychologist.

Alvord, M. K., Zucker, B., & Grados, J. J. (2011). *Resilience Builder Program for children and adolescents: Enhancing social competence and self-regulation—A cognitive-behavioral group approach.* Research Press.

Anderson, R. E., & Stevenson, H. C. (2019). RECASTing racial stress and trauma: Theorizing the healing potential of racial socialization in families. *American Psychologist, 74*(1), 63.

Banks, K. H., Goswami, S., Goodwin, D., Petty, J., Bell, V., & Musa, I. (2021). Interrupting internalized racial oppression: A community based ACT intervention. *Journal of Contextual Behavioral Science, 20,* 89–93.

Bernard, D. L., Calhoun, C. D., Banks, D. E., Halliday, C. A., Hughes-Halbert, C., & Danielson, C. K. (2021). Making the "C-ACE" for a culturally-informed adverse childhood experiences framework to understand the pervasive mental health impact of racism on Black youth. *Journal of Child & Adolescent Trauma, 14,* 233–247.

Bernard, D. L., & Willis, H. A. (2024). Ethnic-racial identity. In W. Troop-Gordon & E. Neblett (Eds.), *Encyclopedia of adolescence* (2nd ed.). Elsevier.

Chorpita, B. F., & Weisz, J. R. (2009). *MATCH-ADTC: Modular approach to therapy for children with anxiety, depression, trauma, or conduct problems.* PracticeWise.

Germer, C., & Neff, K. (2019). *Teaching the mindful self-compassion program: A guide for professionals.* Guilford Press.

Hays, P. A. (1996). Addressing the complexities of culture and gender in counseling. *Journal of Counseling & Development, 74*(4), 332–338.

Hope, E. C., Volpe, V. V., Briggs, A. S., & Benson, G. P. (2022). Antiracism activism among Black adolescents and emerging adults: Understanding the roles of racism and anticipatory racism-related stress. *Child Development, 93*(3), 717–731.

Hughes, D., Rodriguez, J., Smith, E. P., Johnson, D. J., Stevenson, H. C., & Spicer, P. (2006). Parents' ethnic-racial socialization practices: A review of research and directions for future study. *Developmental Psychology, 42*(5), 747.

Jacob, G., Faber, S. C., Faber, N., Bartlett, A., Ouimet, A. J., & Williams, M. T. (2023). A systematic review of Black people coping with racism: Approaches, analysis, and empowerment. *Perspectives on Psychological Science, 18*(2), 392–415.

Johnson, M. M., & Melton, M. L. (2020). *Addressing race-based stress in therapy with Black clients: Using multicultural and dialectical behavior therapy techniques.* Routledge

Malone, C. M., Wycoff, K., & Turner, E. A. (2022). Applying a MTSS framework to address racism and promote mental health for racial/ethnic minoritized youth. *Psychology in the Schools, 59*(12), 2438–2452.

Metzger, I. W., Anderson, R. E., Are, F., & Ritchwood, T. (2021). Healing interpersonal and racial trauma: Integrating racial socialization into trauma-focused cognitive behavioral therapy for African American youth. *Child Maltreatment, 26*(1), 17–27.

Neblett, E. W., Jr., Rivas-Drake, D., & Umaña-Taylor, A. J. (2012). The promise of racial and ethnic protective factors in promoting ethnic minority youth development. *Child Development Perspectives, 6*(3), 295–303.

Rathus, J. H., & Miller, A. L. (2015). *DBT skills manual for adolescents.* Guilford Press.

Sellers, R. M., Smith, M. A., Shelton, J. N., Rowley, S. A., & Chavous, T. M. (1998). Multidimensional model of racial identity: A reconceptualization of African American racial identity. *Personality and Social Psychology Review, 2*(1), 18–39.

Siber-Sanderowitz, S., Glasgow, A., Chouake, T., Beckford, E., Nim, A., & Ozdoba, A. (2022). Developing a structural intervention for outpatient mental health care: Mapping vulnerability and privilege. *American Journal of Psychotherapy, 75*(3), 134–140.

Steele, J. M. (2020). A CBT approach to internalized racism among African Americans. *International Journal for the Advancement of Counselling, 42*(3), 217–233.

Stern, J. A., Barbarin, O., & Cassidy, J. (2022). Working toward anti-racist perspectives in attachment theory, research, and practice. *Attachment & Human Development, 24*(3), 392–422.

Turner, E. A., Harrell, S. P., & Bryant-Davis, T. (2022). Black love, activism, and community (BLAC): The BLAC model of healing and resilience. *Journal of Black Psychology, 48*(3–4), 547–568.

Umaña-Taylor, A. J., Quintana, S. M., Lee, R. M., Cross, W. E., Jr., Rivas-Drake, D., Schwartz, S. J., . . . Ethnic and Racial Identity in the 21st Century Study Group. (2014). Ethnic and racial identity during adolescence and into young adulthood: An integrated conceptualization. *Child Development, 85*(1), 21–39.

Williams, M. T., Holmes, S., Zare, M., Haeny, A., & Faber, S. (2022). An evidence-based approach for treating stress and trauma due to racism. *Cognitive and Behavioral Practice.*

Williams, M. T., Metzger, I. W., Leins, C., & DeLapp, C. (2018). Assessing racial trauma within a DSM–5 framework: The UConn Racial/Ethnic Stress & Trauma Survey. *Practice Innovations, 3*(4), 242.

Yosso, T. J. (2020). Whose culture has capital? A critical race theory discussion of community cultural wealth. In L. Parker & D. Gillborn (Eds.), *Critical race theory in education* (pp. 114–136). Routledge.

Index

B

C

D

E

F

G

H

I

T

U

V

W

About the Author

Ryan C. T. DeLapp, PhD, is a psychologist who works with children, adolescents, and adults in New York City and the Washington, D.C., area. He is the founding director of the Racial, Ethnic, and Cultural Healing (REACH) program at The Ross Center. Dr. DeLapp publishes and presents widely on topics related to healing from cultural stress and empowering individuals of color.